A Year in the Village of Eternity

TRACEY LAWSON discovered the joys of the Italian kitchen while teaching English in Tuscany. After graduating in French and Italian, she spent more than a decade as a News and Features journalist with British daily newspapers; later, while Deputy Features Editor of the *Scotsman*, she had responsibility for editing the newspaper's food and health pages. In 2007 she moved to Campodimele, the village that inspired this, her first book. She now divides her time between Italy and the UK.

A Year in the Village of Eternity

Tracey Lawson

BLOOMSBURY

LONDON · BERLIN · NEW YORK · SYDNEY

First published in Great Britain 2011
This paperback edition publushed 2012

Text copyright © by Tracey Lawson 2011
Photography copyright © by Jason Lowe 2011

The moral right of the author has been asserted

Bloomsbury Publishing, London, Berlin, New York and Sydney

Bloomsbury Publishing Plc, 50 Bedford Square, London WC1B 3DP

A CIP catalogue record for this book is available from the British Library

ISBN 978 1 4088 0999 0
10 9 8 7 6 5 4 3 2 1

Typeset by Hewertext UK Ltd, Edinburgh

Printed in Great Britain 2011 by Clays Ltd, St Ives plc, Bungay, Suffolk

All papers used by Bloomsbury Publishing are natural, recyclable products made
from wood grown in well-managed forests. The manufacturing processes
conform to the environmental regulations of the country of origin.

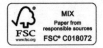

www.bloomsbury.com/traceylawson

For my parents, Joan and George Lawson

To every thing there is a season, and a time to
every purpose under the heaven . . .

ECCLESIASTES 3:1

Contents

The Eternal Table

Come to Campodimele in the spring, in the early morning, when the air is still cool, though the sun is spilling over the Aurunci peaks.

You'll find the village at the end of the mountain road, which twists like a serpent through the wooded crags and the tunnels of newly green trees.

Park up near the statue of San Padre Pio, where the village starts, and if you glance back for a moment the way you came, you'll see the last twists of mist playing on the valley floor.

Now take the fork in the road that leads uphill behind the village – the one where the stone hen houses sprawl. Chances are you'll meet some of the people who feature in this book.

Perhaps Gerardo, zipping past on the aged scooter he's been riding for so many of his seventy-nine years. Or Maria, chasing her hens up the hill on her eighty-three-year-old legs. Or Archimede, who fills his retirement with regular 7 kilometre runs on mountain paths.

Continue uphill and you'll find the eleventh-century walls that encircle the *borgo*, the medieval heart of Campodimele. Ahead is a covered alleyway that cuts through the walls, and if you dip into its centuries-old shadows then out again, you'll emerge onto the old piazza. Here stand houses several storeys tall, reached by staircases made of stone, wreathed in red geraniums which tumble from terracotta pots. Already the front doors are open, and the cooking aromas of garlic, basil and sweet tomatoes are singing on the breeze.

Walk past the house with the mural of the Virgin Mary and follow the curved steps down and round, and below is the main piazza – I think you'll pause at the top of the stone stair to drink in the vista that tumbles off the edge of the square, down to the Liri Valley and towards the Tyrrhenian Sea.

If it's Wednesday, which is market day, you might bump into Assunta, whose brilliant eyes belie her seventy-three years, perhaps buying oranges brought up from the citrus groves of neighbouring Fondi. Or off to forage edible greens in the surrounding fields. Or Adalgesia, for whom market day is more of a social event, because even now, in her seventies, she grows almost all her family's food.

These are just a few of the people I've met in Campodimele, the Italian village that welcomes visitors with a signpost bearing its sobriquet: '*Il Paese della Longevità*', 'The Village of Longevity'.

Others, including scientists and medics, have been known to refer to Campodimele as '*Il Paese dell'Eterna Giovinezza*' – 'The Village of Eternal Youth' – or, as I prefer to think of it, the Village of Eternity.

The reason? The people of Campodimele boast levels of good health and life expectancy which have attracted the attention of doctors both in Italy and further afield.

According to the Comune di Campodimele, 111 of the 671 people who live in the village are between 75 and 98 years old, the age of the oldest person who has residency there. That is to say, 16.6 per cent of the population is over seventy-five, as I write these words. The Commune's most recent statistics, calculated in 2009, find that the average life expectancy of both men and women is ninety-five. That compares to the Italian average of 77.5 years for men and 83.5 years for women, and a European Union average of

75.6 years for males and 82 years for females. Campodimele has been home to an unusual number of centenarians.

It was reports like these which first brought me to Campodimele. At the time, I was a newspaper journalist in the UK, researching an article on foods which might help promote longevity. I kept finding references to an Italian village I had never heard of before.

The more I read about Campodimele, the more fascinated I became. Scientists had found unusually low blood pressure and cholesterol levels in many of its elderly residents; the World Health Organization had investigated the village under the auspices of its Project Monica, which studied communities around the world to monitor trends in cardiovascular disease.

More than these findings, I was intrigued by the descriptions of the villagers and their daily lives. Journalists who visited Campodimele portrayed the elderly residents as unusually vigorous for their ages – pensioners who rode pushbikes, herded goats in the mountains, worked in the fields from dawn 'til dusk, growing almost all their own food. Reporters told how octogenarian men whiled away sunny afternoons playing cards under the elm tree in the piazza while their womenfolk gathered at the hen houses, collecting their suppers of freshly laid eggs.

Levels of heart disease, obesity and cancer were, I read, relatively low in Campodimele.

These people, it seemed, could not just expect to live lives longer than many in Europe. More significantly, in my opinion, they appeared to be able to look forward to a healthier and more active old age than many people in the UK.

Reading about Campodimele from the chaos of my city-dwelling commuter's life in the UK, I longed to sit on the village piazza, sipping espresso beneath its 300-year-old elm tree, enjoying something of the lifestyle which helps these people live so well.

Because, as the Irish satirist Jonathan Swift once wrote, 'Every man desires to live long, but no man would be old.'

And so, in the autumn of 2006 I jumped on a plane to Rome and drove 160 kilometres south along the breakneck *autostrada* and the squiggly mountain roads of Lazio to investigate for myself.

I knew so little about the village then. Situated midway between Rome and Naples, it was about thirty minutes from the coast, in the province of Latina. Teetering on a promontory within the Aurunci Mountains National Park, it was 647 metres above sea level. This much I'd gleaned from the local council's website.

The rest of my imaginings were inspired by my youthful travels in the north of Italy and that peculiar brand of romanticism with which the English view Italian life – a gilded vision of pastoral utopias and culturally rich cities fuelled by the writings of E. M. Forster, D. H. Lawrence and Goethe. The village's very name is evocative – it derives from the Latin *campus mellis*, 'field of honey', for this is the region which cultivated the bees that brought honey to the tables of the Roman Empire.

Arriving in Campodimele, I did indeed discover the archetypal Italian rural idyll: a cluster of stone houses perched high on a sundrenched mountain top; narrow, winding streets encircled by turreted medieval walls; an eleventh-century church with a soaring bell tower; and a piazza with a truly breathtaking panorama across the valley below. And, all around me, evidence of what had brought me there – elderly farmers clambering over olive groves; old women mounting ladders to cut grapes from pergola vines; grandmothers striding up steeply stepped alleyways while balancing bundles of kindling on their heads. I also met one gentleman of 103 years, sitting down to minestrone soup for lunch.

Greeting me in his office at the apricot-coloured town hall, Generale Aldo Lisetti, then mayor of Campodimele, told me he believed that various factors support the health and longevity of the constituents, including the pure mountain air and relatively low stress levels of rural life. Perhaps, he pondered, some residents even enjoy a genetic predisposition to long life. But, like all the other villagers I spoke to, he agreed that there is another factor: diet.

'Fresh, seasonal and chemical-free fruit and vegetables,' said Lisetti. 'Only a little meat and fish. And simply cooked at home.' This is the part of the equation that most interested me, the factor that had led me to trip upon Campodimele in the first place: what people here eat.

The question of what Italians eat is one I have been researching for more than twenty years, in the nicest possible way – by living and travelling in Italy, studying the language and cooking its *cucina* in my own kitchen day in, day out.

I fell in love with Italy and all it embodies as a child on family holidays in the north which introduced me to the sky-scraping Dolomites and to languorous, sinking Venice. Even then I knew that I wanted to learn Italy's lyrical language, confident that one day I would sit in one of the tourist-trap cafés of Venice's Piazza San Marco and order coffees and pastries in the Italian tongue. (Aged eleven, I had no understanding of their astronomical price tags.)

My university studies in Italian and French led me to a summer teaching English in Tuscany, and for four months I used my one free day every week to criss-cross its seductive landscape to discover the treasures of Florence, Siena, Lucca and Pisa. The galleries and antiquities of Tuscany, its cypress trees and sunflower fields, need no introduction, nor do its fabulous dilapidated stone villas surrounded by olive groves which have for so long lured Britons to a new life under the Italian sun.

But from the very start of that summer I realized that, fascinating as the grand attractions of Italy are, the incidentals of daily existence here are even more so: the food the Italians eat and the wine they drink; the bars where they swig early-morning espressos and the family trattorias where they dine; the morning markets where they select the freshest fruit and vegetables for lunch and the *alimentari* still found on every corner, where you can buy the finest cheeses, salamis, olives and bread, to throw together a light evening meal. Of course it wasn't long before I realized that such things are not incidental at all – they are the very essence of the Italian way of life, the foundations upon which an Italian's day is structured; the heartbeat so integral to their soul that Italians struggle to understand any other way of living and eating.

Even in an age in which Italy is ranked as one of the richest and most commercially sophisticated countries on the globe, many of its cities and citizens still find time to take two hours for lunch. And whether at home or in restaurants, Italians demand and receive the best of ingredients, often served in the simplest way, which allows the integrity of each flavour to shine through. I never cease to marvel at the simple delights of Italian cuisine. The way a few slices of plum tomatoes and *mozzarella di bufala* can be transformed into a meal fit for the gods with just a splash of olive oil, a sprinkling of fresh basil leaves and a twist or two of black pepper. Serve this classic salad with a chunk of wholewheat bread and a glass of red wine, and you have a meal as nutritionally balanced and health-giving as you could hope for. And it takes about five minutes to make.

This simple philosophy of marrying the freshest seasonal ingredients with the simplest preparation has informed my entire cooking repertoire over the past two decades. But the merits of the Italian kitchen aside, I know that its place in my heart is also due to the fact that it marries so well with another long-standing interest of mine: the role of food as preventative medicine, and the health merits of the southern Mediterranean diet.

I have no scientific training and I am neither a doctor nor a nutritionist. I profess only a keen layperson's interest in nutrition, fuelled by an instinctive belief that a focus on nourishing our bodies with the right foods is a far more logical way to achieve a healthy body and weight than being obsessed with quick-fix fad diets. And while there is little – if any – evidence to suggest that chemical-light organic foods are better for us than non-organic foods, it has always made perfect sense to me that minimizing the chemical load in our food chain must be better for our health than adding to it through industrial growing, processing and conserving methods.

This uncomplicated way of thinking is born of my experiences in Italian kitchens, where they have a term for such food: *cibo genuino*. Although this phrase renders into English as 'genuine food', I don't believe that those two little words even begin to convey what *cibo genuino* means to people in Campodimele.

For *cibo genuino* is an all-encompassing philosophy – a regard for food that requires that produce is grown, harvested, prepared and served with respect for every link in the chain: the land, the produce itself, the people who eat it and the wider environment.

Such food is ideally grown with zero chemical input, harvested at the peak of perfection, eaten locally, fresh and simply prepared. Preferably eaten in season, it can also be eaten out of season and is still considered *cibo genuino* so long as only natural, or non-chemical, methods of preservation are used: salt, sugar, oil, vinegar; freezing, home-canning or vacuum-packing.

In short, *cibo genuino* is the antithesis of the ready-meal, E-number-rich culture which has such a stranglehold on the everyday eating habits of so many people in the industrialized West, and which is believed by many to be contributing to high levels of heart disease, obesity, diabetes and cancer here.

In Campodimele the way of eating is the epitome of *cibo genuino* – just as it has been for centuries. Many people here still *fanno il contadino* – that is, they retain the small-holding traditions of peasant farmers, to a greater or lesser degree. For many that means a large *orto,* a vegetable garden, adjacent to their homes, where they grow seasonal fruit and vegetables all year round while holding down full-time jobs in spheres unrelated to agriculture. Others, including many retired people, *fanno il contadino* on a full-time basis – growing wheat for bread, keeping a goat for cheese, cultivating a vine-covered pergola for wine; sowing, reaping and raising almost everything which comes to their tables.

Nearly all of this food is produced and eaten just as it has been for hundreds of years: on land fed by natural animal fertilizers and without the use of pesticides. It's picked daily or weekly by hand and eaten within hours of harvesting, so retaining most of its vitamin and mineral content. And it's prepared quickly and simply – grilled, fried, boiled or eaten raw. Seasonal gluts of fresh produce from the *orto* see housewives embark on marathon preserving sessions, to ensure nothing goes to waste. Aubergines are bottled *sott'olio*, in oil, sweet peppers in vinegar; fruit is turned into jam; conserves are put up on the shelves of *cantine* and *magazzini*, the cellars and storehouses that are integral to the cyclical patterns of the agricultural and culinary year here.

To what, if any, extent do the purity and range of foods eaten here contribute to the enviable well-being and long lives of the Campomelani? It is not possible to quantify.

Pietro Cugini, Professor of Internal Medicine at La Sapienza University of Rome and Academician of Lancisi's Academy in Rome, has carried out several studies into the health of the Campomelani. He has tested the biological rhythms and blood pressure of three generations of longevous families, and examined lifestyle elements like their working and walking habits. His studies also cover meal timing – the regular schedule typical of many rural cultures – and dietary habits, such as the intake of macro- and micro-nutrients, salt intake, consumption of coffee and alcohol, of the entire population, from ten-year-olds to those aged over one hundred.

Professor Cugini believes that genetic traits account for 30 per cent of their long life expectancy. The remaining 70 per cent can be attributed to several other factors – their lifestyle and its strong synchronization with the geophysical cycles (rising at sunrise, retiring at sunset); plenty of physical activity into old age; a fair climate amid the Aurunci Mountains, free of air pollution; and of course their diet of 'genuine' foods and their nutritional habits. All of which results in blood pressure significantly lower than the Italian average.

It is impossible to quantify the role food plays in longevity, but Professor Cugini describes the Campomelano diet as *iper-mediterraneo* – hyper-Mediterranean. That is, it exemplifies a diet widely regarded as one of the healthiest in the world, the Mediterranean diet now being recognised by UNESCO as part of humanity's cultural heritage.

The Campomelani eat lots of legumes – beans and pulses such as borlotti, chickpeas, *cicerchie*, a small pulse particular to the area, and *scalogno* (*Ascalonia caepa*), a variety of onion, very rich in antioxidant agents, that was imported by ancient Romans from the city of Askhelon in Israel. Known in Italy as *la carne dei poveri*, 'the meat of the poor', beans and pulses are high in protein, but free of cholesterol, which can harm cardiovascular health.

The scarcity of bovine products in the Campomelano diet is also significant, says Professor Cugini. Campodimele is mountain territory, ideal grazing for goats and sheep, but not best suited to cows. Therefore, beef and butter, which are relatively high in saturated fats, have traditionally featured minimally in the kitchen here. Meat is more likely to come from the chickens that many families keep for eggs and whose flesh is both lean and relatively low in cholesterol, thanks to the freedom these birds enjoy to wander the roads and hillsides. Boar and hare, which live wild in the mountains, are also brought to the table by hunters, and again are relatively lean meats.

Professor Cugini points out that the Campomelani eat a relatively large amount of fish compared to most mountain communities, thanks to the village's proximity to the Tyrrhenian coast – *pesci azzurri*, 'azure fish', as the Italians romantically refer to the schools of oily fish that include sardines and anchovies. These are rich in the omega-3 fatty acids linked to protecting heart health.

The level of salt in the diet is relatively low – just 4 grams daily as opposed to the 6 gram daily allowance recommended by many Western health authorities. High levels of salt and its constituent, sodium, in the diet are of course associated with high blood pressure, which can increase the risk of heart attack and stroke.

And naturally the Campomelano diet is rich in two other elements synonymous with the delights of the Italian table: extra-virgin olive oil, which is rich in monounsaturated fats, and locally made red wine, which is rich in polyphenols, may both protect the heart. Professor Cugini has also found that the drinking of coffee, wine, beer and hard liquors is very limited, as are smoking and the eating of sweets.

In short, if we were setting out to design a diet to promote health and longevity using foods widely available in the Western hemisphere, it might well resemble the eating habits of the Campomelani. Their meals typically begin with the *primo*, the first course, of carbohydrate-rich egg-free pasta called *laina*, often simply dressed with oil and vegetables, followed by the *secondo*, the main course, of protein-rich beans or pulses, fish or lean chicken, along with the *contorno*, the vegetable side dish – perhaps wilted leafy greens, peppers or aubergines. The main course is always followed by *insalata*, salad, to cleanse the palate – perhaps a simple green salad just minutes out of the *orto* – and then cheese, perhaps ricotta made from the milk of mountain goats or *mozzarella di bufala* produced in the nearby towns of Itri, Lenola and Fondi. Then fresh fruit, eaten as it was on the plant, and, on special occasions, a little *dolce*, or sweet. All accompanied by moderate amounts of red wine, and cooked not in saturated animals fat, but in olive oil.

But while the merits of the Campomelano diet are evident, there is no denying that many other factors contribute to health and longevity here.

Professor Cugini points out that the tendency to work the land means that people lead, and have traditionally led, lives which are extremely physically active – a factor which he says is without doubt important to good health.

And elderly people here continue to live sociable lives, many enjoying the support of extended families and the easy day-to-day contact afforded by a small, close-knit community, an active church and a sunny climate, which encourages outdoor activity and that quintessentially Italian social activity – the evening *passeggiata*, a stroll around the piazza. Experts are increasingly recognizing the role of active social structures in the promotion of a healthy old age.

Professor Cugini also believes that some inhabitants of Campodimele benefit from a genetic predisposition to longevity, a conclusion he reached after leading a study into blood pressure patterns among elderly residents, their children and their grandchildren. This study was undertaken as part of his collaboration with the project From Womb to Tomb undertaken by Professor Franz Halberg of the University of Minnesota. Having monitored the blood pressure of more than ninety elderly villagers over a twenty-four-hour period, Professor Cugini found that the mean level in older people was comparable with the healthy levels seen in much younger people. Their progeny too had remarkably healthy blood pressure.

Professor Cugini's fondness for Campodimele and its people is obvious from the way he talks about their easy sociability, their wonderful *cucina* and their *disponibilità* – their willingness to help those keen to study their way of life. He points out that there are many communities across the globe which boast longevity levels higher than that of Campodimele, but that the village is ideal as a model because such a high proportion of its residents share a homogeneous lifestyle, including diet.

It is this which still fascinates me – what people here eat. And while it is true that I was first attracted to Campodimele by its sobriquet of '*Il Paese della Longevità*', it is not the dietary statistics that fuel my love. My heart sings in celebration of the abundance and lush quality of its produce, the simple logic of its seasonal eating patterns and the simplicity with which food here is prepared.

All this, coupled with the beauty of the landscape and the overwhelming generosity and warmth of the people, led me to come and live in this village, in the hope of documenting its agricultural and culinary year. In doing so I have come to fully understand the value of living a seasonal life – a notion of which I was barely even conscious after decades spent living in cities and shopping in supermarkets. And while it is easy to appreciate this in a community whose rhythms are dictated by the agricultural and religious year, I have come to believe that much of what I have experienced here could be transferred to urban life outside Italy – especially at the table. If this is not by growing our own food then it can be by sourcing organic produce, eating fresh what is in season now and preserving seasonal gluts in natural ways to enjoy in the year ahead; by respecting the rightful place of food in our lives, not as perfunctory fuel, but as a keystone of well-being and pleasure; and by carving out a sense of perspective from the blurred momentum of city living by taking time to pause and celebrate food on a monthly, weekly, daily basis – not just the major religious festivals, but the little *sagre*, or thanksgivings, of the table: the excessive lunch of Carnival, the meat-free days of Lent, the first cherries of spring,

December mandarins – often grown far from city streets, but a reminder that Nature's cycle moves on; that everything passes.

I came to Campodimele hoping I might learn how to live longer, but discovered something much more important – how to live well. In doing so, I have been privileged to enjoy the friendship and hospitality of many people. I would like especially to mention Generale Aldo Lisetti, Paolo Zannella and Roberto Zannella – successive mayors of Campodimele – and the current deputy mayor, Alessandro Grossi (who was, in fact, born in England to Italian parents). The unstinting hard work of the men who have led the administration of the Comune di Campodimele and their devotion to the place have helped bring it to the attention of the world. To accept a stranger such as myself into their village demanded great trust and generosity.

The book is not the story of a single chronological year, but a collection of tales gathered over almost three years. It has only been possible thanks to the unlimited kindness and helpfulness of all of the residents of Campodimele – the *contadini* who showed me how they work their land, and the women who flung open their kitchens and larders, who invited me to their tables with a trust and hospitality which I found truly overwhelming. I hope that the people of Campodimele see their beloved village truly reflected in these pages, and that in the stories I have written about them they see themselves. I can never thank them enough for what they have given me – their extraordinary recipe for a long and well-lived life.

Tracey Lawson

2010

January

The Tree of Life

This is where it all begins. In the olive groves, on the mountain slopes, in the first days of the new year.

January is newly born and so much of the landscape seems without life: the black, sodden soil; the snow-sprinkled peaks; the charcoal fingers of trees scratching the metallic sky.

The wind has spittle on its breath, which whispers of a storm tonight, and up on its mountain top Campodimele is hunkering down. Tiers of ochre- and apricot-hued houses huddle around the grey stone church. Its eleventh-century walls hug tight its historic heart. There are no lights in the windows yet, no plumes of smoke on the early-afternoon air. At this hour, in this season, it looks like a village lost in sleep, waiting for a thousandth winter to pass.

But down here, in the olive groves, all is vibrant life. The trees are flurries of silver-green swirls, glistening as they dance with the wind. The olives are purple jewels, ripe and swollen with oil.

More than any other fruit, the olive speaks of the sun: lazy lunches under shady pergolas on balmy days in southern climes; afternoons at tables piled high with food preserved in, bathed in, cooked in olive oil – baby artichokes bottled in oil in the spring, roasted red peppers swimming in green-gold pools, fresh egg frittatas with their oil-crisped crusts. Dishes brought to life by the oil of the olive for these quintessentially Italian meals, which mark leisurely Sundays, family celebrations, *sagre* on summer days.

But for the people of Campodimele, those meals, those sun-drenched moments, start here. Amid the chill of winter, on the mountain terraces, as they bring the olive harvest home.

'*Niente medicinale,*' says Maria, stroking a hand down a feathery olive bough and cupping a cluster of the amethyst-tinted fruits in her hand. There are 'no medicaments' used here, she is saying, no chemicals on these plants.

We're in her olive grove in the Aurunci Mountains, beneath Campodimele's walls. Afternoon is galloping towards night, chased by clouds from the east, but the olive-pickers are working on.

This is the fifteenth day of Maria's olive harvest, she tells me, and there are a further ten to go – more, if time is lost to rain. A month in the field, in the coldest season, one of the toughest tasks on the land. But it's a task for which Maria's family gathers every year, because no harvest is more important than this one. The oil from these olives will be the base note of every dish Maria creates in the twelve months to come. Cooking medium, flavouring, preservative – it will breathe life into the vegetables she grows, the animals she raises, the wild game her menfolk hunt.

Maria stoops to scoop a handful of fallen olives from the ground-net and studies them, her patterned headscarf flapping in the gusting wind. Then she smiles – a smile that glistens in her eyes, as if she can tell already that this year's oil will be particularly good, that she'll enjoy working with it.

'*Un anno sì, un anno no,*' she says – 'one year yes, one year no'. Olive trees bear fruit only every second winter. So you need trees which give olives this year, others twelve months from now, if you want an annual fresh supply of oil.

Michele's late father planted this grove over fifty years ago, carving tiers from the chalky rock with his bare hands. Today three generations of the old man's descendants harvest his legacy: Michele and Maria, their children, Pasquale and Assunta, Pasquale's wife, young Maria, and Assunta's daughter, Michela.

In some ways the harvest is going on as it has for centuries. The women laugh and chatter as they comb the lower boughs with hand-held rakes to bring the olives cascading down. They scoop them into little sacks which Michele straps to his mule, still the only transport that can negotiate the terraced hillside. But new technology is making inroads here. Above the chatter of the leaves comes the whine of the *motorino*, an electric rotor blade which Pasquale is trying out for the first time this year, to strip the highest boughs.

And now, further up the mountain, you can see Michele calling the *frantoio*, the olive mill, to see when this batch can be pressed – his mobile in one hand, his braying mule in the other.

The olive groves end here. Scramble further up the slopes and there are forests of oak, a little snow in the colder months. Squiggle down the mountain along the snake-twist roads, and you'll come to the Tyrrhenian Sea. Campodimele sits 647 metres above those turquoise waters, half an hour inland by road. And this is why the olive oil of Campodimele is so fine.

'*Isolati*,' Paolo di Fonzo says of the Campodimele olive groves, 'isolated' – just like the medieval heart of Campodimele when it was first settled. The circular walls of its *borgo* afforded protection from attack. And the closest settlements are several kilometres away.

Today these factors conspire to protect Campodimele's olive groves from a modern-day pest: *la mosca dell'olivo*, the olive fly. The cool, dry air is unattractive to this insect, whose larvae feed on the olive fruit and have been known to ravage crops in warmer areas. Should *la mosca* take hold in the hotter coastal towns, the undulating landscape of the Aurunci Mountains and its wind patterns offer a natural barrier to its path.

'*Campodimele è un'oasi*,' says Paolo. The village is an oasis for olives. This is why olives here can be grown *senza trattamenti*, without chemicals. Just a handful of growers feel the need to use such sprays, according to Paolo, who is president of the Associazione Laziale Frantoi Oleari – the Lazio Olive Millers' Association. And those who do, he believes, act out of precaution rather than real need.

Just as important to the quality of the oil are natural animal fertilizers, preferably derived from the growers' own livestock.

These factors combined render the oil of Campodimele as pure as can be. I want to use the word *biologico*, 'organic'. But *biologico* is the norm here, so normal that it's a term I never hear in Campodimele. The people here have another word to describe their produce: *naturale*.

Maria has invited me into her *cantina* – that room in the Italian home which is part larder, part storage area: cool and dark in the summer heat, dry and sheltering in the winter months. The olive harvest is in, and the oil has been extracted at the mill. A leg of prosciutto hangs from a beam to air-dry. Red wine slumbers in glassy-green bottles. A silvery vat dominates one side of the room. Michele bends to open its tap and the olive oil flows like liquid light into the *cantina* gloom.

The decanted oil spills down the neck of a glass bottle to smother my fingers. It tastes like the scent of the mountains on a warm summer's day – fruity, grassy, perhaps a hint of herbs. It's the colour of the Aurunci too – green underlaid with sun-faded yellow. Its taste is strong, distinctive, so much so that it will add flavour to every dish, working as an ingredient in itself, not simply as a cooking medium. It is all extra-virgin – oil with an acidity content of less than 1 per cent, the finest accolade any olive oil can receive.

Maria and Michele's families have been cultivating olives on these hills for centuries, she tells me, and I realize that every winter's harvest, every splash and drizzle of oil on pan and plate, is a direct link to the generations who have gone before; a golden thread winding down the years, binding them to a tradition older than memory itself.

There's another sentiment at play here too, that of *cibo genuino*, 'genuine food' produced with respect for the land on which it grows, the animals from which it comes and the unfathomable hand of Nature. '*Tutta roba nostra*,' says Maria, casting a hand around the *cantina* – and this is another phrase you hear here daily: 'All our own things'.

Maria and Michele work the land year-round to produce almost all their own food. The *orto* behind their house has trees bearing figs and walnuts. Their *terreno*, their land, brings tomatoes, peas and beans, onions and potatoes. They keep hens for eggs and raise a pig and rabbits for meat. On the flat belly of the valley they grow wheat to grind into flour for Maria to turn into bread. And on the mountainsides, olives for oil.

Naturale. Cibo genuino. Roba nostra. These are the key principles of food and cooking in Campodimele. To respect them is to understand the wealth they bring to the kitchen – and to accept that the month-long olive harvest, in the grip of winter's breath, is no hardship after all.

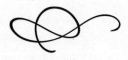

Olivi ai finocchietti — Olives with wild fennel seeds

Wild fennel grows in the hedgerows of Campodimele, and its seeds offer a sweet foil to the saltiness of olives. The crushed seeds are very pungent, and a few go a long way.

Two or three handfuls of cured green olives
Four large cloves of garlic, peeled and squashed by the side of a
    knife
Few pinches of wild fennel seeds, lightly crushed
Few pinches of crushed dried red chilli
Good splash of extra-virgin olive oil

Place all the ingredients together in a bowl and mix well.

Leave to marinate for at least twelve hours, stirring frequently, then serve at room temperature as antipasti.

Insalata condita – *Classic Campomelano dressed salad*

A plate of fresh green salad leaves is eaten at almost every meal in Italy – after the *secondo* and before the cheese and fruit. Instead of mixing the dressing before adding it to the greens, as the French often do, Italians simply splash the ingredients directly onto the leaves. This reflects the simplicity of the Campomelano *cucina* – a dash of oil, vinegar and salt, a little adjustment to taste, and *pronto*.

Handful of green salad leaves per person
Extra-virgin olive oil
White-wine vinegar
Fine sea salt

Wash the salad leaves and use a salad-spinner to remove excess water – too much water clinging to the leaves will prevent the dressing penetrating the greens.

Place the leaves in a bowl, then pour over a few splashes of olive oil – enough to lightly coat the leaves.

Next, splash a few drops of vinegar onto the salad, followed by a scattering of salt.

Mix gently until the dressing is well distributed, and taste – add more of any ingredient, according to preference.

Pinzimonio —
Raw vegetables dipped in olive oil
and other condiments

Barely a recipe, this is a wonderful informal start to a dinner with family and friends which, like so many Campomelano dishes, requires minimal preparation.

Selection of raw seasonal vegetables such as celery, carrots, red and
   yellow peppers, and spring onions
Small vessel of extra-virgin olive oil
Small vessel of white-wine vinegar
Salt cellar filled with fine sea salt
Small dish of crushed dried red chilli

Slice the vegetables into small batons and lay out on a serving dish alongside the containers of olive oil, white-wine vinegar, salt and chilli.

Invite each diner to place a little of each of the condiments on their plate, then to choose a selection of vegetables and dip them one by one first into the oil, then into the vinegar, salt and chilli on their plate, according to preference.

A Pig for All Seasons

'You feed a pig for a year and then you kill it,' says Leana, swiping a hand across her throat. 'Then the pig feeds *you* for a year.'

The balance to this equation, the unsentimental logic in these words, epitomizes the Campomelano approach to food: the understanding that as much as you put in, you will get out; the acceptance that *ogni cosa ha il suo momento* – everything has its time.

It's the end of January, one of the coldest days of the year so far, and in the phase of *la luna calante*, the waning moon – three elements which, when they coincide in Campodimele, traditionally signal the time to kill the family pig.

'When I was little I used to ride the pig like a horse,' Leana recalls. 'Then my father would kill it, under the archway, in the street outside this house. I was always sorry to see the animal die – but what could I do? Then we'd clean it, hang it, cut it up and – *salsicce*.'

Salsicce, the Italian for 'sausages', and the Campodimele term for sausages made from raw meat and then air-dried. *Salsicce* are among the most prized of Campodimele's *caserecci* foods, that is to say foods produced *a casa*, at home. In this first week of the waning moon, some households have already slaughtered their home-reared, acorn-fed pigs in just the way Leana remembers. They are salting the hind legs as the first step to making air-dried prosciutto, and curing the underbelly to create fat-streaked *pancetta*. But animals take time and space to keep, and today many families no longer raise a pig, sourcing their meat instead from producers they trust. But they still insist on making and preserving their *salsicce* at home.

This is what we are doing today: Leana, Irma, Adelia, Assunta, Margherita and me. Leana's house snuggles halfway up a stone staircase built into the village walls. Her husband, Gerardo, was born in this house, and it has been in his family for more generations than he can count: people have been making air-dried sausages in this kitchen for hundreds of years.

The making of this year's batch began last night with the delivery of the meat. The weather has been perfect this past couple of days: cold enough to ensure the pork can be hygienically handled; dry enough to ensure the raw meat won't be ruined in too-damp air.

The meat arrived in huge chunks, carrying plenty of fat, to keep the sausage moist and flavoursome. Leana diced the 50 kilos into 1 centimetre cubes then mixed it with traditional spices. *Peperoncino*, hot chilli pepper, is the key seasoning in these parts, where black pepper has yet to make inroads. *Petartela* in Campomelano dialect signifies dried, crushed coriander seeds, used by the ancient Romans to preserve meat. '*A chi piace*,' says Leana when I ask how much of each spice is added per kilo of meat: 'As you wish.' I hear this phrase often, and at first I find it incredibly frustrating – how to recreate the wonderful flavours of these kitchens without precise measurements of the herbs and spices used in each dish? But soon I realize how liberating it is – every cook in every home is making every dish to their own taste, or that of the family they cook for. There is seldom a right or wrong amount – just a rough indication of how much according to personal preferences and availability.

So Leana has added *peperoncino* and coriander seed *all'occhio*, which is to say by eye. When pressed, she describes the amount as '*un bel po*', 'a good bit'. These are two more non-specific measurements of the kitchens of Campodimele. However the one for added salt is precise – 30 grams per kilo of pork – because salt is added not just as a flavouring but also for its vital preservative powers.

After marinating overnight, the pork is ready, and a good glass of white wine is added for every 10 kilos of meat, to prevent the *salsicce* drying out too much. Irma has carted her *salsiccia*-making machine across the rain-splattered piazza and up the stone staircase to Leana's house. It's a metal cylinder with a nozzled end which rests on a red-enamelled frame complete with a hand-crank. And so the sausage-making can begin.

Margherita is washing the animal intestines, which will serve as the sausage casings, slipping the ends of the milky-white metre-long tubes onto the tap and allowing water to course through them. Leana and Irma stuff the cylinder with the chopped, seasoned meat and lower it onto the red frame. Adelia slips one end of the intestine onto the nozzle and ties a piece of string around the other end. Irma turns the crank and the pork slips through the nozzle and into the casing. As it emerges, Leana stabs the sausage at intervals with a safety pin, to expel trapped air. When the intestine is filled, Assunta holds the sausage while Adelia cuts lengths of string and ties it at intervals.

Leana is making 50 kilos of sausages: 15 kilos for her own family; 5 for Adelia's daughter; 20 for Gigino, whose daughter, Gina, is married to Leana's son, Nino; and 10 for another friend. She has already made the *salsicce al fegato* from pig's liver and other offal; this sausage, prized as a local delicacy, is increasingly hard to come by. Each of today's batches is tied with a different colour of string, because each is made with a different mix of spices, *a chi piace*.

'*Siediti*,' says Leana, 'sit down.' She guides me to a seat by the stove. Then she chucks a handful of diced pork into a small frying pan, stirs it and tips it out onto a plate. '*Buona per sale?*' she asks, handing me a fork. 'Enough salt?'

The meat is tender, plump and juicy to the bite, spicy with the heat of the *peperoncino* and a faint background note of coriander and plenty of salt. A glass of red wine appears from nowhere, and now Leana is taking a knife to a loaf of bread she has made with wheat flour from her own fields and baked in her wood-fired oven. '*Mangia, mangia!*' she urges, the phrase epitomizing Italians' endless hospitality: 'Eat, eat!'

But these sausages are not destined to be *salsicce fresche*, the fresh sausages made the same way but cooked and eaten immediately. These are to be air-dried then preserved *sott'olio* and eaten over the next twelve months.

In the past, such methods of preservation were a matter of necessity and survival – a way to preserve the various cuts of the precious pig when meat was a rare luxury, but a valued source of protein. Today it is a matter of choice, driven not by some romantic notion of maintaining a tradition but by the desire to eat chemical-free foods, *cibo genuino*.

Leana balances a blue plastic bowl of sausages on her head and beckons me up a flight of stone stairs to another small kitchen then heads back downstairs for more sausages. A whittled branch is suspended horizontally from the ceiling, and it's from this that the sausages will be hung. The corner fireplace, set with branches to be lit, will house a low flame almost constantly for several weeks to ensure the air is dry enough to cure the sausages, but not so hot as to ruin them. The faint aroma of wood-smoke will permeate their animal casings.

I'm wondering how many kilometres of sausages have dried in this room over the centuries when I hear a metallic clanging. Leana and Assunta are lugging a 2 metre aluminium ladder up the stone stairs. Assunta is seventy-three, Leana seventy-six, and I'm little more than half their age, but it would not occur to them to ask me to help. Moments later, Leana is climbing the ladder and stringing up another batch beneath the ceiling. Then Gerardo, two years older than her, takes her place, hanging length after length of *salsicce* over the branch. After hanging, the sausages will be preserved in jars filled with olive oil and stored in cool, dark cellars.

The whole process requires three to four weeks, but little hands-on time. But for the next twelve months four families will have an instant supply of pork meat in their store cupboards. It will be sliced and served as antipasti or added to *ragù*, delicious mixed-meat sauces. Leana will ask Gerardo to pop down to the cool darkness of their *cantina* and bring up a jar of *salsicce* to fry up with leafy green *broccoletti* as a quick and simple dressing for pasta. A kind of fast food, slow style, I think, as he hangs the last of the sausage, descends the ladder and prepares to light the drying fire.

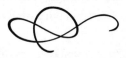

Salsiccia piccante – Air-dried spicy sausage

Air-drying sausage is a time-honoured art and requires key factors to prevent the sausage going rancid and to avoid the risk of food poisoning. All equipment and surfaces must be sterilized, and the pig-intestine casings must be procured from a reliable, hygienic source. The sausages must be made in cold conditions then air-dried for several weeks in a room that is cool, free of damp and aided by a constantly lit wood-burning fire.

This recipe makes eight sausages, but if you are going to the trouble of procuring pig intestines and a sausage-stuffing machine and air-drying your own sausages, it's well worth making five times that amount and preserving some in oil.

1 kg (2lb 3oz) mixed pork and pork fat – around 70 per cent
     meat, 30 per cent fat – roughly chopped
1 scant tsp ground hot chilli pepper
1 scant tsp ground coriander
30g (1oz) fine sea salt
50ml (2fl oz) good dry white wine
2m (7 feet) cleaned pig intestines or synthetic casings, cut into
     70cm (2 foot) lengths for ease of handling
2m (7 feet) fine kitchen string, cut into lengths of around
     15cm (6in)
A sausage-stuffing machine or a wide-nozzled piping bag
Metal skewer

The night before you want to make the sausages, mix the pork meat and fat with the chilli, coriander, salt and white wine. A quantity of 30g (1oz) of salt per kilo of meat may seem a lot, but the salt plays an essential role in preserving the air-dried sausage, so don't skimp, and ensure it is well distributed among the meat. Cover and leave to marinate overnight for at least twelve hours in the fridge.

The next day, mix well to ensure the ingredients are evenly distributed.

Place the lengths of pig intestine in a large bowl. Take a length from the bowl and insert a funnel into one end of the tubular intestine, then pour 2 litres (4 pints) of cold water through the intestine, discarding the water that exits at the other end. Run your fingers along the intestine to drain as much water as possible. Repeat with the other lengths of intestine.

Now tie a length of string around one open end of each intestine, so sealing it. If you have a sausage-stuffing machine, fill with the meat mixture according to the manufacturer's instructions, and proceed to stuff the intestines. If using a piping bag, attach one end of an intestine length to the piping nozzle, fill the bag with meat, and proceed to stuff the intestine, pushing the meat mixture down towards the sealed end as you go. Repeat with the other intestine lengths; as you stuff, you might find it useful to prick the filled skins at intervals, using the metal skewer (or a wooden cocktail stick) to eliminate air bubbles. As the intestines fill up, use string to tie them into sausages every 12cm (5in) or so, and tie the loose end with string too.

When all the meat has been made into sausages, suspend the links in a cool, dry room with an open hearth. Light the hearth fire using only wooden kindling – if you have oak logs, so much the better. The fire should smoulder, filling the room with smoke to help flavour the sausages, and create a warm room to dry them. The fire should burn constantly throughout the period during which the sausages are drying – usually three to four weeks.

First-hand experience is the best way to tell if the sausages are dried. They should be shrunken, the skins wrinkled, the meat inside firm, with a glassy finish when cut. How long they take to cure will depend entirely on the original moisture content of the meat and the thickness of the sausages.

Air-dried sausages can be eaten immediately – sliced as antipasti or even as a *secondo*. They will keep well wrapped in greaseproof paper in the fridge for a week or two, but will continue to dry out, so eat them quickly.

Excess sausage can be preserved *sott'olio*. Thoroughly sterilize and dry a lidded jam jar large enough to hold two or three sausages, place them in the jar then fill it to the top with olive oil, firmly secure the lid, and store in a cool, dark place until needed. Well-cured sausages can keep like this for up to a year.

Makes around eight sausages.

Salsiccia fresca piccante alla brace –
Fresh spicy sausage over charcoal

This is sausage made with the same ingredients as those used for air-dried sausage, but is designed to be cooked and eaten straightaway. Because it is not preserved, and because pork is naturally quite salty, it requires just a fraction of the salt needed for the air-dried version. In Campodimele it is often prepared *alla brace*, grilled over the embers of a wood fire – the forerunner of modern-day barbecuing.

One quantity of sausages made according to the recipe for air-dried sausage on page 30, but instead of using 30g (1oz) salt, use just a few good pinches to taste

If you are lucky enough to have an open-hearth fire, an hour or so ahead of serving, set some branches to burn and allow them to reduce to charcoal. If you are using a barbecue, prepare it according to the manufacturer's instructions.

Place the *salsicce* in a barbecue pan, set to cook, and turn frequently until cooked through.

Makes around eight sausages.

February

The Mountain Gives You Everything

La montagna ti da tutto. The mountain gives you everything.

This is a phrase you hear often here, but I'd lived in Campodimele a long time before I fully understood what it means. In every moment, in every season, the mountain provides all the things you really need; the very essentials of life.

In days gone by, this peak offered protection, which is why Campodimele was established here. Walk the circle of its eleventh-century defensive walls, counting twelve watchtowers as you go, and you will have the medieval watchman's view.

And the mountain forests offer fuel – oak and beech to fire the ovens and stoves on which so much food is still cooked here. And there's water too, in the low-lying wells that served the village before these modern days.

The Aurunci also give their settlers space – grassy slopes on which to graze goats and sheep. Land to carve into olive terraces, or flatten into fields for wheat.

Even uncultivated, the mountain is replete with food: leaping hare and wild boar in the colder months; spring strawberries and autumn mushrooms; thyme and mint, wild fennel too, to flavour food; or chamomile to help you sleep. Seek and the mountain will give.

'You just need to know where to look,' says Assunta as we slip down the slope by her rickety little hen house at *le galline*, the sprawl of outhouses behind the village where the hens live. But really it's a question of knowing *how* to look – once you learn to read the mountain flora and fauna, you can see that food is everywhere.

I've been to Assunta's hen house more times than I can remember, in every month of the year, but it's only these past couple of weeks that I've spotted the thin, green, jagged-edged leaves we're picking today. In January I must have trampled them underfoot. They were just one more bit of green on the hill. Little did I realize that they were *verdure* – edible leafy greens.

The word *verdure* derives from *verde*, 'green', and while it's used as a general word for vegetables, it serves most commonly as the umbrella term for the cooked leaves so frequently served as a *contorno*. The variety of *verdure* is endless here, and every season has its signature greens, some grown in the *orti*, others gathered wild.

In spring the fields are lush with *caccialepre*, *pilosella* and *crispino*, wild leaves and grasses whose names defy translation and which are gathered by hand to boil with potatoes for the wonderfully named *patate pazze* – 'crazy potatoes'. In summer the *orto* has spinach and *scarola*, the prickly, bitter lettuce that is the classic green to add to pans of minestrone soup.

But it's as the weather cools that *verdure* dominate the landscape. The kaleidoscope that was the summer *orto* fades, leaving only deepest shades of green. Autumn brings the first of the *broccoletti*, not broccoli but leafy turnip tops also known as *cime di rapa* or *rapini*, as well as *bietola*, swiss chard and *cavoli neri*, the black cabbages that perch like random sculptures in near-nude fields.

The cold weather also brings the leaf we are looking for today.

'*Cicoria!*' says Assunta, wrenching the leaves from the soil. Chicory, though these leaves bear no resemblance to the pale yellow Belgian endives also known as chicory in the UK.

In years gone by, when money was scarce, wild plants and animals were key supplements to *cucina povera*. And even though times are much better, many villagers forage or hunt for food just as they always have done.

'Because it's there,' says Assunta, employing the classic phrase a climber might use to explain why he would climb the Faggetto, the snow-sprinkled peak that rises behind Campodimele.

Little by little, Assunta has taught me to read the mountain greens. It was she who first told me about *tagne*, the Campodimele frittata fashioned from a particular kind of wild leaf mixed with a little flour, olive oil and salt. Italian frittatas usually contain eggs, omelette-style, and their absence from this dish is evidence of how poor those who once lived on *cucina povera* truly were.

My education in greens began one May morning, during my first spring here, when I joined the villagers on their annual pilgrimage to La Civita: the sanctuary of La Madonna della Civita that sits high on one of the Aurunci peaks, 14 kilometres from Campodimele. We set off on foot at 6.00 a.m., the air still cool and damp, streaking with mist as the heat set in. As we headed downhill I heard the thudding of feet behind me and turned to find Assunta running to catch up. She was mentally totting up how many times she'd made this pilgrimage on foot – sixty, maybe more – when she plunged off the road and into the undergrowth. '*La tagne!*' she exclaimed, snapping a skinny green string of a climbing plant which I later discovered to be *Clematis vitalba*, or 'old man's beard'. Said to be toxic in large quantities, a little, well-cooked, appears to be fine.

Assunta told me she had more *tagne* at home. Would I like to try some? And so, after we'd walked 14 kilometres to La Civita, after the celebration of the Mass, and after we'd hitched rides home, she made me one of the frittatas I'd heard so much about. She simply washed the *tagne* greens, boiled and drained them, chopped them roughly, laced them with olive oil and a little salt, and folded in a little finely ground flour. She flattened the mixture into a skillet and fried it *piano, piano* – gently, gently – and we ate it hot and crispy, its grassy herb flavour like nothing I had ever tasted before.

The *cicoria* we are seeking today are leaves Assunta has gathered all her life. They are only just ready, she tells me, young and tender, so they'll taste bittersweet. She slips them into one of the plastic carrier bags everyone seems to carry in case of a fortuitous roadside find, then she shrugs. That's it. All that remains is to clean the *cicoria* leaves and boil them in salted water until the stalks are soft to the bite. Assunta will drain the *cicoria* then toss it in a frying pan in which she has heated a little olive oil and allowed some squashed garlic cloves to chase their juices. She'll sprinkle a pinch of *peperoncino* onto the greens, and the hot chilli pepper flakes will sparkle like jewels against the dark green leaves.

We head to her house on the piazza of the *centro storico*. And we eat the greens – after the *primo* of spaghetti in her home-conserved tomato sauce – alongside the *secondo* of beef fillets fried in olive oil.

Assunta pours me some mineral water from a plastic bottle and remembers how, as a little girl, she would walk 2 kilometres to Pozzo della Valle, the shepherds' settlement behind the village, to draw water from the wells then carry it home in a two-handled terracotta *pignatta* jug balanced on her head. I ask her again about recipes for mountain-hare stew and wild boar *ragù*, at one time the only source of meat for many locals.

And we reflect on how the mountain has provided our lunch today. Just as it has always given the people of Campodimele what they need.

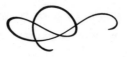

Spaghetti con broccoletti, aglio e peperoncino — *Spaghetti with broccoletti, garlic and red chilli*

Broccoletti are not broccoli, but leafy turnip tops – known as rapini in the US. The leaves are best boiled, but the tiny florets are also delicious pan-fried, as this brings out their almondy taste. If you can't find *broccoletti*, try tiny heads of purple sprouting or tender-stem broccoli instead.

400g (14oz) dried spaghetti
Three or four good splashes of olive oil
Two large cloves of garlic, finely chopped
Two handfuls of small broccoletti florets, washed
Crushed dried red chilli
Fine sea salt

Bring a large pan of salted water to the boil, add the spaghetti and cook it according to the instructions – usually eight to ten minutes.

A few minutes before the spaghetti is cooked, heat the oil in a large, deep frying pan and gently fry the garlic for one minute. Add the *broccoletti* heads and cook for a further two minutes, stirring constantly, and ensuring the garlic does not brown. Add a few pinches of hot chilli.

When the pasta is al dente, drain it and add to the pan of garlic and *broccoletti*. Remove from the heat, and stir, ensuring every strand of pasta is coated in the sauce.

Serve immediately in warmed bowls.

Serves four.

Cicoria con olio e aglio —
Chicory greens with olive oil and garlic

Garlic-infused olive oil is a standard dressing for cooked *verdure* of all kinds here — chicory greens, as in this recipe, spinach, swiss chard, *broccoletti* or *cavolo nero*. The Campomelani sprinkle hot chilli pepper over the cooked, dressed leaves, or in winter, a squeeze of lemon juice from fruit picked that very day in the citrus groves of Fondi.

1kg (2lb) chicory greens — or other leafy greens — washed
    and trimmed, tough stalks discarded
Three or four splashes of olive oil
Four or five cloves of garlic, peeled and squashed by the side
    of a knife
Crushed dried red chilli or juice of quarter of a lemon (optional)
Fine sea salt

Bring a large pan of salted water to the boil, add the leaves and boil for around seven minutes until cooked.

Meanwhile, gently heat the oil and garlic in a large, deep pan, so that the garlic chases its juices into the oil.

Drain the cooked leaves into a colander and squeeze out as much water as possible.

Use two forks to gently separate the leaves, then tip them into the pan of oil and garlic and toss well.

Sprinkle with the chilli or the lemon juice, if desired.

Serves four.

Tagne — *Green frittata*

First forage your *tagne*! But be sure you have identified your finds correctly, to avoid poisoning yourself.

Four or five large handfuls of tagne greens
Few splashes of extra-virgin olive oil
Fine sea salt
3 tsp '00' Doppio Zero flour or plain finely ground flour

Wash the *tagne* greens, discarding the toughest stalks.

Bring a large pan of salted water to the boil and simmer the greens for around ten minutes until tender.

Drain through a colander, refresh the greens with cold water then squeeze out as much water as possible. With a clean, dry tea towel, pat away any residual moisture.

Place the greens in a large bowl, and toss them in a couple of good splashes of olive oil and a pinch of the salt.

Sift in the flour then toss the greens, flour-coating them.

Heat a splash of olive oil in a small non-stick frying pan then add the greens, flattening them with a spatula. Fry them gently on a low heat for around five minutes.

When the underside of the frittata is golden and crispy, flip it over in the pan. To do this, remove the pan from the heat, place a large plate over the frittata, invert the pan so the frittata falls onto the plate then slide it back into the pan.

When the underside is ready, tip the frittata onto a plate. Allow it to cool then slice into wedges.

Serves four to six.

Patate pazze — Crazy potatoes

This wonderfully named dish is a classic of *cucina povera*, using greens which grow wild on the mountains to flavour potatoes which may be past their best after more than six months languishing in the *cantina*.

1 kg (2lb) potatoes suitable for boiling — all of a similar size
Selection of wild mountain greens, such as caccialepre, pilosella,
    crispino or chicory greens (not Belgian endive)
Three or four splashes of extra-virgin olive oil
Three or four cloves of garlic, peeled and squashed by the side
    of a knife
Fine sea salt

Fill a large pan with cold salted water. Scrub the potatoes clean, but leave their skins on, and add to the pan of cold water. Cover, bring to the boil, and let the potatoes cook for around ten minutes.

Add the washed and trimmed greens to the pan, and continue to cook until the centres of the potatoes are soft to the point of a sharp knife.

Remove from the heat and drain through a colander. Separate the greens and squeeze out any remaining water.

If preferred, slip the potatoes from their skins then slice them roughly, combine again with the greens, and place on a warm serving dish. Add the olive oil and the garlic, and sprinkle with salt. Serve warm.

Serves four.

Carnival

Once, this was the only way. To mix your hen-fresh eggs into fine-ground flour by hand; to knead and knead until the two become one; then to roll and roll until the yellow sheet is so spare that the sun shines through it as you lift and flip it in the early light.

Watching Natalina work her fresh egg pasta, it's incredible to think that at one time this ritual was played out in every kitchen here, almost every day. Once for lunch, perhaps again for dinner, on a cold winter's evening.

On most of those days gone by, in most homes, the pasta dough would have been simpler than this – just flour and water, because eggs were too valuable to lavish on pasta at every meal. It would have been mixed and flattened and sliced by hand into ribbon-like *laine* and served dressed with cooked beans: *laine e fagioli*, the signature pasta dish of Campodimele.

On special days, *cucina povera* might be enriched by *pasta all'uovo* – fresh pasta made with eggs. Perhaps cut into thick strips of *pappardelle* to eat with the first wild boar stew of the hunting season. Or sliced into stringy *tagliolini* and cooked in a *brodo*, or broth – if a hen could be spared for the pot. Or flattened thin, thin, thin, then cut into rectangular leaves and interlaid with thick slicks of meat sauce to create perhaps the most famous *pasta all'uovo*, which is what Natalina is making today: lasagne.

'*Carnevale, Pasqua, Natale*,' says Natalina, draping her pasta dough over her rolling pin, scattering her board with flour, laying the pasta flat and rolling again. Carnival, Easter, Christmas Day. These are the religious festivals at which lasagne is traditionally consumed in Campodimele, days of thanksgiving and celebration or, as in the case of *Carnevale*, a determination to *carpe diem* – to seize the day – as my friend Pietro loves to exhort us to do.

Seizing the day is, I am realizing, an essential component of life here, because, as the *contadini* say, '*Ogni cosa ha il suo momento*' – everything has its moment. If it's sunny today, it's the moment to sow your fields, because if it rains tomorrow you won't be able to. If the crop is ripe, harvest it now, or it will spoil on the plant. Because Nature and the weather will have their way, and to live well from their fruits, you must dance to their rhythms.

Italian *Carnevale* is the spiritual and culinary incarnation of this philosophy. Carnival may be synonymous around the world with the masked spectacular played out on the waterways of Venice, but in fact it is the Christian festival that falls on the Tuesday before Ash Wednesday – that is, the start of Lent, the forty days leading up to Easter Saturday. In this predominantly Catholic country, many still observe Lent as a time of penance, to commemorate Jesus's forty-day fast in the wilderness. Traditionally, those who could afford meat renounced it at this time, hence the term *Carnevale*, derived from the Old Italian phrase *carne levare*, 'the removing of meat'.

With forty lean table days ahead, the day before Lent has evolved as a *carpe diem* day of excess, thus *Carnevale*'s alternative name of *Martedì Grasso* – Fat Tuesday, a direct equivalent of the better-known French term *Mardi Gras*.

Not so long ago, there was *fame*, hunger, in Campodimele, as in so many rural parts of Italy prior to the post-war boom years. '*Si capiva niente di lasagne*' – 'We knew nothing of lasagne' – say many of the older villagers of this import from the north. Now times are better, the days of hunger are gone, and lasagne has also emerged as a traditional *Carnevale* dish here – rich egg pasta, richer meat sauce, combined in a dish that serves only as the first course of a sumptuous meal. One *Carnevale* lunch I enjoyed lasted seven courses and what seemed as many hours: antipasti of prosciutto and *salumi*, followed by the lasagne *primo*, then a *secondo* of *salsicce* simmered in white wine and served with *broccoletti*. Then a palate-cleansing green-leaf salad, followed by cheese, then fruit, and finally *struffoli*, the little fried *Carnevale* cakes. So much last-ditch feasting that as my pudding *prosecco* sparkled on my lips, the prospect of forty lean lunches ahead seemed like a blessing, not a penance.

But making fresh pasta limits your opportunity to seize the day, I think, as I watch Natalina at work; little chance to step out into the *orto* to harvest the tomatoes to add to your meat *ragù*; little time to tend the hens who lay the eggs with which *pasta all'uovo* is made.

Natalina drapes her pasta over the rolling pin again and, placing her floured hand in its centre, smooths the dough towards the edges of the wooden shaft, first to the left then to the right, before dropping it onto the table top and rolling it again, to within a few millimetres of its existence.

She created this pasta by cracking eggs into a pile of '00' flour, Italy's famous *Doppio Zero*, 'Double Zero'. Although some families still grow their own wheat for bread, shop-bought '00' seems to be the most popular choice when fresh *pasta all'uovo* is called for. It's fine-ground and sieved not once, but twice by the miller, hence the '00' tag. It creates a strong, smooth, elastic dough that is resistant to tearing. Ideal for the wafer-thin lasagne leaves Natalina is now cutting into rectangles and dropping into simmering water, a splash of olive oil in the pan to ensure they don't stick together.

It's taken her half an hour, perhaps longer, to bring her pasta to the *punto giusto*, 'the right point'. I imagine the Campodimele kitchens of generations gone by, before dried packet spaghetti became the workaday norm. Hand-making the basic *laine* for families of six, seven, maybe more: grandparents, cousins, an uncle or two, hungry from working in the fields. Wherever did women find the time?

And why do they still take the time to do this now? Dried pasta can be found in most kitchens here these days, but freshly made *pasta all'uovo* is frequently on the table now that higher living standards mean the meat sauces which accompany them are more affordable.

'*È un'altra cosa,*' Natalina says of her fresh egg pasta when I comment on the time and effort it takes and the packets of dried lasagne leaves sitting on shelves in nearby shops. Her response is a familiar one. Literally, it translates as 'It's another thing'. But these words, usually said with a shrug, have connotations of 'It's a better thing', 'It's a more genuine thing' and, of course, 'It's a tastier thing'. Dried, shop-bought pasta is welcome because it is quick and convenient and will free you to leave the kitchen and make the most of a suddenly sunny winter's day. But '*Se vuoi mangiare meglio, devi fare così*' is another familiar mantra of this place. 'If you want to eat better, you have to do this.'

The *ragù* for the lasagne is bubbling on the stove. It's a rich red sauce that sings of summer tomato vines, springtime onions, white wine. And *vitello macinato*, minced veal, a meat that was once rare in the *cucina povera* of Campodimele, if available at all in the hardest times: a rich treat for *Martedì Grasso*. Natalina has added a handful of sweet green peas to her *ragù*, grown in her summer *orto* and then frozen. '*A chi piace,*' she says – as you like it. There are no rules to *ragù*; every cook makes it her own way.

As Natalina prepares to layer the lasagne, I realize something is missing. To me lasagne is a trio of elements – layers of yellow pasta interlaced with meat *ragù* and milky, buttery béchamel sauce. The last of these, *besciamella* as the Italians call it, is not here.

'*Niente besciamella*,' confirms Natalina. Flinging open her oven door, she whips out a ceramic dish alive with a bubbling, hissing mass of lasagne. The *ragù* runs like lava as she parts the pasta layers with a fork to reveal something white, creamy, molten beneath – *fiordilatte*.

Fiordilatte, 'flowers of milk', is the romantic name for the soft, round spheres of cow's milk cheese also known as *mozzarella per cucinare*, 'mozzarella for cooking', because it resembles buffalo mozzarella, but has a drier texture.

Cheese instead of *besciamella*. This, I learn, is a common way of making lasagne here, although other Campodimele cooks insist on home-making *besciamella*. I can't help feeling that lasagne without *besciamella* is a reflection of how cooks adapt imported dishes to their own terrain. *Besciamella* requires cow's milk and butter, but this is mountain territory, best suited to grazing for goats or sheep. Lasagne is a johnny-come-lately dish here, and when it arrived, it would have been easier and cheaper to use what was home-produced. Perhaps this is why cheese became the third element – in the past, goat's or sheep's cheese, perhaps that day's newly made ricotta, or the firm rolls of fresh *formaggio*, or maybe a handful of matured, dried pecorino, grated and scattered over the *ragù*.

Cheese is not really a substitute for *besciamella* in lasagne, but rather *un'altra cosa*. Even melted, its consistency is thicker, creamier, and that's ideal, because around here, as in most of Italy, a good lasagne should have a firm, almost solid structure, the sauce spare and just moist amid the pasta, not lavish or wet. Eating Natalina's lasagne is like sinking your teeth into a *millefoglie* pastry – layer upon layer of corn-yellow pasta baked to an al dente firmness punctuated by melted cheese soft against the textured meat of the *ragù*, pasta which encourages rather than overwhelms the appetite ahead of the rich main course. A world away from the floppy, sloppy lasagne I have so often encountered outside Italy.

Now that transport links are better, the dairy ingredients of *besciamella* are easily available, but this habit of cheese remains in many homes – after all, why spend half an hour blending flour, butter and milk when *fiordilatte* can be sliced and scattered in the space of a moment? When you have fresh *pasta all'uovo* to hand-make? And another day of your life to enjoy?

It's some time after *Carnevale* that I realize why *lasagne all'uovo* is the perfect *festa* dish. That it can, in fact, save you time. I have guests coming to lunch tomorrow, and pasta for ten to cook, and I doubt even my biggest pan has space enough to boil a kilo of dried spaghetti. However do people cater for those huge gatherings of family and friends, the frequent religious *feste*, the string of saints' days?

Lasagne. Trays full of it. Half an hour mixing the pasta, but no more than an hour for the *ragù* to cook, less than an hour in the oven. Also, I'm assured, lasagne made today and allowed to relax overnight will taste even more delicious reheated tomorrow. One less dish to prepare *al momento*, 'on the day'.

So I make my lasagne in the cool gloom of the morning, as the orange fingers of daylight come beckoning across the mountain tops. Crack eggs from my neighbour Maria's corn-fed, walkabout hens into a kilo of *Doppio Zero* flour. Knead the dough by hand then roll it flat, flat, flat on my marble worktop, before holding it up to delight in the shafts of sunlight shining through.

A little later, once it's cooked, I can be sure that we'll eat well tomorrow. And that I can leave my kitchen to seize this morning on the mountain, to make the most of what Nature offers today.

Lasagne al vitello macinato – Lasagne with minced veal

In Campodimele, many home cooks insist that savoury dishes should use either onion or garlic – never both. However some cooks accept that the two can work well together and unless you can access the freshest, tastiest organic ingredients, you might find the inclusion of garlic in this recipe helps. If you don't have time to make your own pasta, this recipe also works well with good-quality dried egg lasagne.

For the pasta:
500g (1lb 2oz) '00' Doppio Zero flour or plain white flour, plus
    extra for dusting
Four medium-sized organic eggs – as fresh as possible
or 500g (1lb 2oz) dried egg lasagne, preferably organic

For the ragù:
Two splashes of extra-virgin olive oil
Two medium golden onions, finely chopped
Three large cloves of garlic, peeled and squashed by the side
    of a knife (optional)
400g (14oz) minced veal or lean minced beef
Two or three good pinches of fine sea salt
Two glasses of good dry white wine
1 litre (2 pints) conserved tomato sauce (see page 263)
Handful of fresh or frozen peas
200g (7oz) fiordilatte mozzarella, thinly sliced
Freshly grated Parmesan to serve, if desired

First make the pasta.

Tip the flour onto a large, flat surface or into a large bowl, and create a well in the centre – if you are using plain flour instead of '00', sieve the flour.

Crack the eggs into the well and break the yolks with your fingers. Keeping your thumb static in the centre of the egg mixture, use your fingers to gradually draw small amounts of flour into the eggs, mixing the two together well before drawing in more flour.

Continue until the flour is incorporated into the eggs, mixing for longer and longer periods as the pasta comes together – this will take some time.

Once you have drawn the pasta together into a ball, lightly dust a large, flat working surface with flour, place the pasta on it, and begin to knead it: use the heel of your hand to push the part of the pasta nearest to you down and into the body of the pasta, then pull the part farthest away up and backwards towards you, then repeat the kneading process. Continue until the pasta is firm, but elastic – this may take around twenty minutes. Slick a tiny amount of olive oil on your hands if you find the pasta sticking during kneading.

If you have time, cover the pasta with a clean, damp tea towel and allow it to rest in a cool place for half an hour.

Now start the *ragù*.

In a broad-based, deep pan, heat a couple of splashes of extra-virgin olive oil. Add the onion and the garlic (if using) and fry gently over a low heat for a few minutes.

Next, add the minced meat to the pan and use a wooden spoon to break it up into small chunks. Continue to move the meat around the pan for a few minutes until it is browned on all sides and chasing its juices.

Add two or three pinches of fine sea salt, to taste.

Cook for a few minutes more to allow some of the juices to evaporate. Add the wine and cook for a further few minutes, until the alcohol has evaporated.

Next, add the tomato sauce and the peas, if using fresh ones. Bring to the boil and allow to simmer for twenty to thirty minutes, stirring frequently, until most of the liquid has evaporated. If using frozen peas, add them now.

Preheat the oven to 200°C/400°F/Gas Mark 6.

When the pasta has rested, cut it in half and lay one half onto a floured work surface. Be sure to keep the other half wrapped in the damp tea towel to avoid it drying out.

You now need to roll the pasta as thin as possible without tearing it. To do this, use a long rolling pin to flatten it, then lift and turn the pasta through 90 degrees before rolling again. Continue rolling and turning until the pasta thins – at this point it may be easier to turn the rolling pin rather than the flattened pasta. Two or three times during this process, gently roll the pasta onto the floured rolling pin, reflour the work surface, and roll the pasta back onto the work surface, the other side down.

When the pasta is around 3 to 4mm (⅛in) thick, roll it onto the pin and hold it up to the light – if you can see the light shining through it, it's ready. If not, roll it a little longer until it does.

When the pasta is thin enough, and the *ragù* is ready, bring a large pot of salted water to the boil and add a splash of olive oil.

Cut the pasta into rectangles which measure roughly 15 by 10cm (6 by 4in) to create the lasagne leaves. Drop two or three leaves of lasagne into the pan of boiling water, allowing them to cook for a couple of minutes or so.

While the lasagne leaves are cooking, slick around a quarter of the sauce over the bottom of a large lasagne dish.

After two minutes, use tongs to remove the lasagne leaves from the pan and place them over the sauce in the dish. Cook more leaves until the first layer of sauce is totally covered by lasagne leaves. Then slick another quarter of the sauce over the lasagne leaves in the dish, and cook more lasagne leaves to create a second layer of pasta.

Spoon over the third quarter of the *ragù*, and place a few slices of the *fiordilatte* or other cheese on top of the sauce, followed by a third layer of lasagne leaves made from the ball of reserved pasta.

Place most of the remaining *ragù* on top, reserving a few dessertspoonfuls, then place the remainder of the cheese on top of this.

Now add the final layer of pasta, and scrape the little bit of remaining sauce over the top.

Use a metal fork to prick several holes through the layers of pasta, before placing the lasagne in the oven for around forty minutes.

In this part of Italy, lasagne should have an almost solid structure, emerging in firm bricks when cut – not the sloppy, unstructured lasagne so often served outside the country. If it looks a little runny, cook for another ten or fifteen minutes with a sheet of aluminium foil placed loosely over the dish to prevent burning.

After removing from the oven, cover with foil and allow to rest for fifteen minutes in a warm place before serving. It will taste even better reheated the next day. Serve with freshly grated Parmesan, if desired.

Serves six.

Pappardelle al ragù –
Fresh egg pasta ribbons with meat sauce

Every region of Italy has its own version of *ragù*, and, within that region, every city, town and village will make *ragù* with distinctive characteristics – usually dictated by what animals and *odori* are local to the area. This recipe includes the three classic *odori* used in Campodimele: onion, celery and flat-leaf parsley. The meat is cooked in large chunks so it can be eaten as the *secondo* after the juices have been used to dress the *pappardelle* and eaten as the *primo*. This means that both courses are cooked at once.

For the pappardelle ribbons:
One quantity of fresh egg pasta dough, as per the recipe for
  lasagne on page 51, or dried egg pappardelle if you don't
  have time to hand-make the pasta

For the ragù:
One large golden onion
Two small sticks of celery
Large handful of fresh flat-leaf parsley
Three good splashes of extra-virgin olive oil
800g (2lb) selection of chunked meat: pork shoulder, off the bone;
  beef – topside or chuck are perfect for stewing; salsiccia fresca,
  made to the recipe on page 33 or shop-bought – use spicy or
  non-spicy, according to preference
Two glasses of good dry white wine
1.5 litres (3 pints) conserved tomato sauce (see page 263)
Two or three good pinches of fine sea salt (optional)
Handful of fresh basil leaves, torn

If making the pasta by hand, first start cooking the *ragù*, and make the pasta while the *ragù* is cooking.

To make the *ragù*, finely chop the onion, celery and flat-leaf parsley – if you have one, use a *mezzaluna*, the half-moon-shaped, two-handled knife whose curved blade makes quick work of chopping.

Heat the olive oil in a large, deep pan then add the chopped *odori*, cover with a lid, and fry gently over a low heat for around ten minutes, stirring occasionally until the onion is translucent but not brown.

Add the pieces of meat to the pan and allow them to fry gently in the *odori* for five to ten minutes; this helps the meat take on the flavours of the *odori* and seals it. Make sure the *odori* do not burn, as this will ruin the *ragù*.

When the meat is lightly browned on all sides, add the wine and turn up the heat, simmering the meat until the wine has reduced by about half and the alcohol has completely evaporated.

Then lower the heat and simmer the *ragù* very gently, covered, for one to two hours until the meat is cooked through, but still tender – the length of time it requires will depend on the size of the chunks of meat.

About forty-five minutes before the *ragù* is ready, add the tomato sauce, stir well, and cook for a further forty-five minutes or so, until the meat is fork-tender.

Once the *ragù* is ready, taste and add salt, if required.

While the *ragù* is cooking, make the fresh egg pasta, according to the instructions in the recipe for lasagne on page 52. Cover with a damp cloth and allow the pasta to rest for around half an hour.

Once the pasta has rested, divide it into two, leaving half wrapped in a damp tea towel.

Now roll out the pasta until it is just 3 to 4mm (⅛in) thick at most – using the method described in the lasagne recipe. Roll it into a shape which is as square as possible then dust the top surface with flour.

To make the *pappardelle*, take the far edge of the pasta, gently roll it towards the centre, and stop. Now take the near edge and roll it towards the centre – you should end up with pasta in the shape of a snail with two tails.

Now use your sharpest knife to cut the pasta into *pappardelle* about 1.5cm (½in) wide, slicing through both 'tails' simultaneously.

Unravel the pasta ribbons, dust lightly with flour so they don't stick together, and place them on a large tray. If you are preparing the *pappardelle* in advance, cover them with a damp tea towel to prevent them drying out.

Unwrap the reserved half of the pasta and create a second batch of *pappardelle* in the same way.

Next, add the torn basil to the pan of *ragù* and stir to ensure it is distributed throughout the pan. Now remove the pieces of meat from the *ragù* and place them on a warm serving dish, leaving the juices and small flakes of detached meat in the pan.

Now bring a pan of salted water to the boil, and cook the *pappardelle* until they are al dente – this is likely to take anything between three and five minutes, depending on the thickness of the pasta, and the only way to be sure is to bite into a piece of *pappardelle* out of the pan every thirty seconds or so when you think it is nearly cooked.

When the *pappardelle* are ready, drain through a colander, but do not shake dry, or they will stick to one another.

Now tip the *pappardelle* into the pan of *ragù* juices, stir gently, and serve the coated *pappardelle* in bowls as a *primo*.

The reserved chunks of meat and sausage can be served afterwards as the *secondo* – the idea is that everyone should have a little taste of each kind of meat in the pot. If dining more informally, among family, it's more usual to serve the *secondo* meat and sausage at the same time as the dressed *pappardelle*, for ease.

Because this recipe contains onion, many Campomelani would not dream of adding garlic to the mix. However, if you prefer to do so, or if you are unable to procure the tastiest organic vegetables, you can add three large cloves of peeled garlic crushed against the flat blade of a knife when you add the other *odori*.

Serves six.

Tagliolini in brodo — Tagliolini strips in chicken broth

This is another example of two-dishes-in-one cooking. The boiled chicken flavours the first course of *pasta in brodo*; then the chicken is eaten separately as a second course.

For the tagliolini:
One quantity of fresh egg pasta (see page 51)

For the brodo:
Slick of extra-virgin olive oil
One large golden onion, very finely chopped
Small handful of fresh flat-leaf parsley, chopped
Two sticks of celery, crushed, plus their leaves, finely chopped
One large carrot, cut into quarters
Two cloves of garlic, peeled and squashed by the side of a knife
*   (optional)*
Fine sea salt
200ml (7fl oz) conserved tomato sauce (see page 263) or four
*   fresh plum tomatoes, skinned and deseeded*
One large potato, whole
One whole, organic free-range chicken, skin discarded

Heat just a little olive oil in a pan large enough to hold the chicken along with enough water to cover it.

When the oil is hot, add the onion, parsley, celery and its leaves, carrot, garlic (if using) and a good pinch of salt, and gently fry them for up to five minutes, without colouring.

Add the tomato sauce or fresh tomatoes, if using, and the potato, then bring the pan to a simmer.

Add the chicken and enough cold water to completely cover it, about 1.5 litres (3 pints), to the pan.

Bring to the boil, lid the pan, lower the heat, and allow to simmer for one and a half hours. Every so often skim off any scum which rises to the surface, and top up with a little hot water to ensure the chicken remains covered.

Now make the fresh egg pasta. Cover it with a damp cloth and allow it to rest for around half an hour.

Once the pasta has rested, divide it into two, leaving half wrapped in a damp tea towel.

Now roll out the pasta until it is just 3 to 4mm (⅛in) thick (see page 53). Roll it into a shape which is as square as possible then dust the top surface with flour.

Take the far edge of the pasta, gently roll it towards the centre, and stop. Now take the near edge and roll it towards the centre, making a snail shape with two tails.

With a sharp knife, cut the pasta into *tagliolini* 3 to 4mm (⅛in) wide, slicing both 'tails' simultaneously.

Unravel the ribbons and dust lightly with flour.

Unwrap the reserved half of the pasta and create a second batch of *tagliolini* in the same way.

After one and a half hours, pierce the thickest part of the chicken thigh with a meat skewer – the juices should run clear. If not, continue to simmer until they do.

Remove the chicken from the pan, wrap it in foil, and leave it in a warm place to rest.

The liquid remaining in the pan is the *brodo* – the broth. Skim off any scum, remove and reserve the potato, carrots and celery, and taste the *brodo* to see if it has enough salt.

Now bring the pan to the boil again, throw in the pasta ribbons, and cook for around two to three minutes, until they are al dente. If you don't make *tagliolini*, use dried pasta like spaghetti, and cook according to the instructions on the packet, usually about eight to ten minutes.

Serve the *tagliolini in brodo* as the *primo*. Afterwards serve the chicken, cut into pieces, as the *secondo* accompanied by the carrots, potato and celery and a *contorno* of wilted greens such as *cicoria* (see page 42).

Serves six.

MARCH

Cinnamon Season

Easter smells of cinnamon here. Of aniseed too. One a rich red scent of far-off lands, the other the warm green breath of Campodimele's fields.

You can mark the calendar by the herbs and spices whose smells waft from kitchen windows – a kind of olfactory code by which to measure the months. Coriander signals January and tells you that the *salsiccia* is hanging to dry; mint means May on the mountain meadows, its sweet perfume exploding underfoot; basil speaks of summer, the first hot days of June, or of one of the hotter months to come. Cinnamon and aniseed are the sign that *dolci di Settimana Santa*, sweets for Holy Week, are being made. Chocolate is there too, but not until Easter Day, when every *uovo di cioccolato*, or chocolate egg, must be unwrapped and smashed – a less-than-holy ritual to secure good luck.

It's hard to imagine how cinnamon, an exotic, expensive spice, first found its way up here. From the trees of Oriental forests to this Western mountain top in the hungry days of *cucina povera* – it seems such an unlikely route.

I wonder if it trickled down from Venice, whose merchants once monopolized Europe's spice trade with the East? Or did a peddler bring it up from Naples, where the sweet *sfogliatelle* are made – shell-shaped pockets of feathery pastry stuffed with baked ricotta, cinnamon spice and candied citrus peel? Whichever direction cinnamon arrived from, *torta di ricotta alla cannella* – ricotta-cheese tart flavoured with cinnamon – is, I'm assured, a traditional Easter sweet in Campodimele, strange though it seems to me.

The scent of aniseed is easier to explain – although it's not really aniseed at all. The copy-cat aroma is, in fact, that of wild fennel, which flowers yellow in September, another scent on the breeze which would tell a time traveller who fell to Earth here which season we were in.

'*Papà fa questo*,' says Aminta, whose husband, Roberto Zannella, is mayor of Campodimele. She reaches up to her kitchen shelf and, unscrewing the lid of a glass jar, lets me inhale the scent of dried *finocchietti*, wild fennel seeds: 'My father gathers these.' From the untamed borders of managed fields, the verges of mountain tracks – uncultivated common grounds are a free-for-all larder here, and I too have shaken showers of wild fennel seeds into my cupped palm and carried them home. They are the key flavour in another of Campodimele's signature Easter sweets – *tortano*.

'*Tor-tano!*' is the response I receive when I tell people that I want to make *tortano* at home. The emphasis is correctly on the first syllable, but a note of puzzled exclamation permeates the entire word. *Buono*, everyone agrees – good. But *tanto lavoro* – so much work. All that hand-mixing, then a wait of at least two days for the dough to rise.

I find this response odd. Time spent preparing good food is regarded as an investment in health and happiness here, a duty too. Why this reluctance to make *tortano*, the ring-shaped leavened cake whose texture falls somewhere between sponge and brioche?

I don't have to wait long to discover the problem with *tortano*: it's a capricious cake.

In this village where excellent cooking is the norm, I hear more exasperated stories about making *tortano* than happy ones. It can take up to three days for the dough to rise if the weather is cold, I'm warned, possibly more – *non si sa mai!* You never know!

'It tasted too strongly of yeast,' says a friend famed for her home-baked bread, but who admits to throwing her last batch of *tortano* in the bin. 'The dough didn't rise,' laughs Paulina, Aminta's mother. 'It just wouldn't rise!' This, after revealing that the *tortano* she served me with coffee came from the bakery in nearby Lenola.

My friend Bruno, however, has happy memories of making *tortano* as a child. His mother, Regina, would cook ten in a single batch every Easter, to last the family through Holy Week. They were stored in a *mallia*, a wooden table-cum-storage chest with a flip-top lid, which was where the weekly home-baked bread loaves were kept.

Regina is ninety-eight now, but the recipe for making ten *tortani* trips off her tongue as surely as if she made her last batch yesterday: '*venti uova, 4 kili di farina, 1 kilo di zucchero, 50 grammi di sale*': twenty eggs, 4 kilos of flour, 1 kilo of sugar and 50 grams of salt. Plus, she adds, a little leavening.

She tells me how she would mould the dough into rings, glaze them with beaten egg and shovel them into her *forno a legna*, the wood-fired oven built into the walls of many houses here, the only means of baking before gas and electricity arrived.

'The oven mustn't be too hot,' Regina advises, though how to gauge the temperature of these centuries-old domestic infernos I've no idea. 'And cover the dough with wool, a blanket, until it's risen.'

I often see Regina about the village, especially in summer – she walks with a stick now, but climbs up and down the stone alleys and stairways to attend Mass at San Michele Arcangelo. Sometimes I'll feel a soft hand on my arm as I chat on the piazza, and turn to find Regina pausing to talk during her *passeggiata*. She still sews on a hand-turned Singer sewing machine, which she says is '*più vecchia di me*', 'older than me'. The day she talks to me about *tortano*, she shows me pink bed-socks she has just knitted – fairy-fine stitches woven on sliver-thin needles. And the orange shawl she's crocheting next.

She gave up making *tortano* long ago, though. After all, you can buy good ones today, and most people have the cash for such things, *grazie a Dio* – thanks be to God. I realize that if Regina doesn't recommend making *tortano* at home, then it's not going to be the easiest of tasks.

The cinnamon-spiced ricotta tart is a different matter.

Ricotta is in season in the spring, and this is why it is used in this celebratory sweet. After long, cold, wet winters, the mountain goats and sheep birth their kids and lambs in March and April, and produce copious amounts of milk – enough to suckle their young and for the shepherds to make cheese. First comes *formaggio*, the long cylinders made from fermented milk solids, and then ricotta, which literally means 'recooked': the soft, creamy cheese created from the reheated whey that remains after *formaggio* has been made. Ricotta is at its best in the first few weeks of spring: sweet with the scent of the new mountain grass and tiny flowers on which the animals graze.

We're in Aminta's light and airy kitchen – Aminta, her mother, Paulina, and her sister-in-law, Irma. It's a huge *cucina abitabile*, a habitable kitchen, the term Italian estate agents use to describe a kitchen with room for a dining table and living area – still the most desirable space to have in an Italian home. Irma is passing the ricotta through a *mulino per verdure*, a hand-operated vegetable mill. The ricotta wriggles out of the little holes like creamy spaghetti. Irma beats it into eggs, sugar and a little glass phial of *aroma di limone*, lemon oil, and adds a sprinkling of cinnamon.

While Irma works, Paulina makes the *sfoglia*, the sheet of pastry casing, from flour, sugar, an egg, a pinch of salt, another sprinkle of cinnamon and, to my surprise, olive oil. I've never seen oil used to make pastry before – but then it's the most convenient and cheapest fat in these parts. Today, if animal fat is required even for sweet tarts, *strutto*, or pork lard, is often the choice – a taste dating back to the times when most families raised and slaughtered pigs of their own.

Paulina mixes the ingredients in a bowl, then slams the dough onto the stone worktop and proceeds to break all the rules I ever learned about handling pastry intended to bake to a shortcrust consistency. She kneads the dough vigorously for several minutes, then flattens it as thin as can be with a rolling pin. Then she holds the pastry up towards the kitchen window and smiles as the light shoots through it.

'Like for fresh egg pasta,' says Aminta.

The tart tin is lined with pastry, the ricotta filling is poured in, the pastry trimmings are used to create *strisciarelle,* thin strips laid in a lattice effect on top – and into the electric oven it goes.

There are easier Easter sweets of course – not least the *colomba pasquale*, or paschal dove, a cake baked in the shape of the Christian symbol of new life and peace. Richly textured like the panettone of Lombardy, aviaries of *colomba pasquale* perch beribboned in the shops just now, waiting to be bought by those who have neither the time nor the inclination to bake.

In Campodimele, however, it's still a tradition in many extended families for the women to gather in a single kitchen to create Easter sweets. There are three sweets which traditionally close the Easter Sunday meal. First is *torta di riso*, a rice tart whose filling is a string of imports: rice itself, which must have arrived from the plains of the north because it isn't grown here; cloves, another exotic from the Orient; and lemon rind, brought up from the citrus groves of Fondi, 25 kilometres down the mountain. Second is *tortano* – if it rises to life. And third is *torta di ricotta*, which Aminta is removing from the oven now.

It's spectacular – the ricotta has risen like a soufflé and billows like a cotton-wool cloud gilded by golden sunlight, bouncing on a spring breeze; if not for the latticework of pastry, it would surely float away. Slowly, it comes to ground and, exhaling its heated breath, sinks and settles, perfectly flat. Cold, it tastes sweet and creamy, the cinnamon more subtle to the tongue than to the nose. It's refreshing in its simplicity, perfect as a follow-up to the rich meat stews of a celebratory meal. Though as Aminta removes a second tart from the oven, I think that I'll make it again and again, all year round, simply to see the feather-light milky filling wriggle within its pastry cage, as if trying to escape back to the mountain pastures from where it came.

My kitchen smells of fennel today. It did last week too. And a couple of weeks before that. The *tortano* has worked on this third attempt: rich-textured but spongy, and soft to the bite. It was worth the two days of waiting for the dough to rise – and the two times it didn't before that.

But although the cake has finally come right, it's also wrong, I realize. Because Easter Sunday is well past. We welcomed this key date of the Christian calender in an achingly cold church with Midnight Mass, heating our hands on hand-held candles lit by the paschal flame. And the snow-scorched tips of the Aurunci have once again melted to green. Today, the air is thrillingly hot, calling for the cool notes of mint, the calm breath of chamomile, the sweet, fresh cut of basil through heavy air. Beside them, fennel and cinnamon emerge here as rich, warm scents, perfect for calling you off cold streets to wood-fired hearths.

Ogni cosa ha il suo momento. Everything has its moment. And that for fennel is past, for cinnamon too. Only next Easter will I welcome them back.

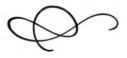

Torta di ricotta alla cannella — Ricotta and cinnamon tart

Italian celebratory cakes are, in my experience, very large — presumably to ensure every member of the extended family who has gathered round the table can enjoy a slice. The recipe below requires a tart tin measuring roughly 27 centimetres (11 inches) in diameter and 3 centimetres (1 inch) in depth. A small *mulino per verdure* is also useful.

For the filling:
Butter, for greasing
800g (2lb) ricotta — sheep's milk ricotta is traditional, though many today use the milder mix of sheep's and cow's milk ricotta that is widely available in Italy
Eight medium-sized fresh organic eggs
8 heaped dsstsp granulated white sugar
Grated rind of one small lemon or one small phial of aroma di limone
1 level tsp ground cinnamon

For the pastry:
200g (7oz) '00' Doppio Zero flour, preferably containing wheat starch, plus an extra dusting of flour for rolling
2 dsstsp granulated white sugar
½ tsp cinnamon
Good pinch of fine sea salt
One medium-sized fresh organic egg
2 dsstsp extra-virgin olive oil
Another egg — to brush the pastry before baking

Preheat the oven to 180°C/350°F/Gas Mark 4. Grease the tin with a little butter, and dust lightly with flour.

If you have a *mulino per verdure*, place it over a large, deep bowl, and pass the ricotta through it, so it emerges like strands of spaghetti. If you don't, make twenty or so vertical incisions into the cheese east–west, followed by twenty vertical incisions north–south, tip it into the bowl, and beat until smooth.

Break the eggs into a separate bowl and beat well. Add them to the bowl of cheese and mix thoroughly, ensuring the cheese blends smoothly into the eggs.

Add the sugar, the lemon rind and the cinnamon to the bowl, and mix thoroughly. Allow to rest.

Now make the pastry by tipping the flour onto a large flat surface, or into a bowl if you prefer. Add the sugar, cinnamon and salt, and mix well. Create a well in the centre of the flour mixture.

Beat the egg mixture again, add the oil, and stir throughly. Pour into the well in the flour mixture.

Using the fingers of one hand like a claw, and starting in the centre of the well, gradually work the flour into the liquidy centre, mixing each addition in properly before adding another handful of flour. Continue until you have a cohesive mound of pastry dough.

Now you need to knead the pastry dough firmly for several minutes – as you would for fresh egg pasta dough. Continue until the dough is smooth and all the flour has disappeared.

Now lightly dust the worktop and a wooden rolling pin with flour, and roll the pastry into a large, thin sheet. To do this, use north–south rolling movements, followed by east–west rolling movements. Then roll the pastry onto the rolling pin, flour the worktop again, flip the sheet of pastry over, and repeat the rolling procedure. Repeat several times, until the pastry is just a few mm (⅛in) thick. Ideally you should be able to hang it over the rolling pin, hold it up to a window, and see the sun shining through it!

When the pastry is ready, carefully line the tin with it, using a sharp knife to cut away any excess. It's vital that the filling does not leak out, so if small tears appear in the pastry, repair them with a bit of the leftover pastry, stuck down with a little beaten egg. Reserve the leftover pastry for the *strisciarelle* pastry strips.

Ladle the ricotta mixture gently into the pastry-lined tin.

Roll the leftover pastry into one long strip, and use a pastry wheel or sharp knife to cut this into six *strisciarelle* long enough to stretch across the tin.

Beat the extra egg well, and brush some of it around the pastry crust.

Place the strips across the surface of the ricotta at intervals to form a diamond-shaped lattice, pressing their ends well down onto the tart crust.

Brush the remaining egg over the *strisciarelle* to add a sheen to the cooked pastry.

Bake the tart on the middle shelf of the oven for around thirty to forty minutes – it's ready when the ricotta has risen like a soufflé and the pastry lattice is golden brown.

Allow to cool in the tin before serving; serve at room temperature, preferably the following day.

To ring the changes, some Campomelani add a dessertspoon of dark chocolate drops to the filling before pouring it into the pastry case.

Serves twelve.

Tortano – Ring-shaped Easter Cake

The method described below finally produced a cake worth eating. If you are able to access *lievito naturale*, sourdough starter, use it in this recipe. If not, you can start your own using the instructions on page 228. It will need a couple of weeks to ferment before you start making the *tortano*.

1kg (2lb 3oz) '00' Doppio Zero flour
Five medium-sized fresh organic eggs
250g (9oz) white caster sugar
12g (½oz) fine sea salt
*One heaped tbsp wild fennel seeds, lightly crushed in a pestle and
    mortar*
Small handful of lievito naturale, chopped into pieces
Extra egg for glazing

The evening before making the *tortano*, mix the *lieveto naturale* in a bowl with around 250ml (½ pint) tepid water, and allow it to ferment overnight.

The next day, place the flour in a large, flat bowl and create a well in the centre.

Beat the eggs in a bowl then add the sugar, salt, wild fennel seeds and starter. Mix well.

Pour the mixture into the well in the centre of the flour, and, using your fingers, gently draw the inner edges of the flour into the mix, combining it well with the wet ingredients. Continue until all the flour is mixed in.

Tip the dough onto a flat work surface and knead it – press the heel of your hand forwards into the edge of the dough nearest to you, then pull the edge farthest from you up and over the rest of the dough towards you, and repeat. Continue kneading for fifteen to twenty minutes, until you have a smooth, elastic dough.

Place the dough in a bowl twice its size, cover with a clean tea towel or cling film, and set aside in a warm place to allow it to rise to double its size – this might take two to three days.

If, like many people in Campodimele, you are lucky enough to have a *forno a legna*, allow it to burn until the branches are reduced to charcoal. Otherwise, preheat your oven to 200°C/400°F/Gas Mark 6.

Now tip the leavened dough onto a floured work surface, and cut into three pieces.

Roll a third of the dough into a thick, long sausage, bring the ends round to meet each other, and fasten them smoothly to create a ring. Do the same with the other two pieces of dough.

Lightly grease three baking trays with olive oil, and position the *tortani* on them. Beat the extra egg in a bowl, and use this to glaze the *tortano* rings.

Bake for around thirty-five to forty-five minutes, until the *tortani* are golden brown on top and a metal skewer emerges clean from the cakes.

Cool on a metal rack, and store in an air-tight container.

Makes three *tortani*.

Torta di riso alla cannella – Rice tart spiced with cinnamon

For a sweeter take on this spiced rice tart, some Campomelani add a dash of Strega herb-infused liqueur to the filling.

For the pastry:
One quantity of pastry made with olive oil, as in the recipe for
    torta di ricotta alla cannella on page 71
One egg to brush the pastry

For the filling:
400g (14oz) riso classico – the classic rice available in Italian
    delis (or use pudding rice)
500ml (1 pint) fresh organic full-fat milk
One large strip of unwaxed lemon rind – be careful to ensure
    there is no pith attached
Three cloves
Five medium-sized fresh organic eggs
200g (7oz) granulated white sugar
1 level tsp ground cinnamon
2 tsp Strega liqueur (optional)

Preheat the oven to 180°C/350°F/Gas Mark 4.

Lightly grease a 27cm (11in) diameter tart tin, and dust lightly with flour.

Make the pastry and line the tart tin according to the instructions on page 72, using the leftover pastry to create six *strisciarelle*.

Heat a large pan of water. Once it is bubbling, add the rice, return to the boil, and simmer for five minutes.

Drain the water from the rice. Add the milk to the pan, along with the lemon rind and cloves, return to the boil, and simmer on a very low heat for five minutes.

Remove the pan from the heat and leave to cool, uncovered, for at least an hour.

When the rice-and-milk mixture is cool, remove the lemon rind and cloves. Beat the five eggs well in a large bowl, and mix in the sugar. Pour the rice into the eggs along with the cinnamon and the Strega liqueur (if using), and mix thoroughly and quickly.

Pour the filling into the pastry-lined tin and position the *strisciarelle* over the surface, pressing firmly down at the edges to hold them in place.

Beat the egg for glazing well in a bowl, and brush it over the *strisciarelle* and the edges of the tart crust to add a sheen to the cooked pastry.

Bake on the middle shelf of the oven for forty to forty-five minutes, until the pastry and rice topping are slightly golden on top.

Serves twelve.

Looking for Mamma

'*Guarda la Mamma!*' Adalgesia di Fonzo points a green-stained finger into the middle distance, sweeps aside the low-hanging branch of an olive tree and repeats the words she has been singing every few minutes for the past hour: 'Look, there's the *Mamma*!'

And now she's gone. Striding up the stony hill path, slithering sideways down the grassy bank, grabbing the roots of an olive tree for support as she leans at a dizzying angle to inspect the spindly, fern-like leaves known hereabouts as *la Mamma*.

'*Dove si trova la Mamma, si trovano gli asparagi,*' she explains – where you find the Mamma, you find asparagus.

And she does. Poking up from the pine-dark leaves of the Mamma, combat green as if hiding from hunters, is the tall, straight shoot and plaited tip of *asparago selvatico*, wild asparagus. A sharp snap amid the spring stillness and the spear is hers, slipped into the bundle of a hundred or so others she has gathered this morning, the centrepiece of today's *cucina*.

Our asparagus hunt began at 7.00 on this spring morning, when the air was still cool enough, the grass still damp enough to keep the snakes in their sleepy hollows. But by 8.00 a.m. the sun is already strong in the sky.

'*Serpenti,*' says Adalgesia, a warning that the grass-green snakes will be stirring along with the rising heat, in search of hot rocks and food. But she is undeterred. She's been hunting wild asparagus for fifty years or so, ever since she married her husband, Elio, and came to live with him in Taverna, the lower fraction of Campodimele which straddles the main mountain road. Aged seventy-three and armed with a sturdy stick, she will require more than the threat of snakebite to keep her from foraging for this springtime treat.

'*Ogni cosa ha il suo momento*,' says Adalgesia. This is the *contadino*'s mantra I now know so well. Either we collect them now or they will be gone.

The wild asparagus season is short, lasting just six to seven weeks in March and April, and this brief window means it is eagerly anticipated. Farmed asparagus is already in the shops, but the delicate flavours of the white, purple and even green cultivated varieties bear little resemblance to the deliciously grassy bitterness that characterizes the wild stuff.

Hence the armies of asparagus hunters to be seen foraging around the hillsides of Campodimele in recent days. They come in many guises – head-scarved *contadine* harvesting their own grassy terrains, middle-aged townies who have parked up their Mercedes to raid common grounds or even the outer edges of someone's land. These latter know they are unlikely to find a single bunch of wild asparagus for sale at a market or greengrocer's, and blessed is the home cook who invites you round to sample their hand-picked spears.

The asparagus hunters are at their most visible the day after rain because wild asparagus loves spring showers: after a few hot, dry days you might find none, but a single decent downpour will send them shooting skywards, shiny and stiff, and this is the moment to pick them, when they are newly sprouted, bursting with bitter juiciness. If you can find them, that is.

This is my first asparagus hunt, and already it feels as if it will take me the whole season to spot just one spear, never mind enough to make the asparagus frittata Adalgesia is going to show me how to cook. The spears grow singly, sparsely, in the shady spots of the olive terraces behind her house. The *Mamma* is not, in fact, the mother of the asparagus spear, but a spear that has gone unpicked and over time transformed itself into a profusion of lacy leaves around 30 centimetres long. The *Mamma* is the best clue to sourcing a freshly sprouted spear, Adalgesia reminds me, but discerning it amid the riot of spring greenery is harder than it sounds. Even once I've found the leafy Mother, I need two or three minutes of scanning her foliage and a lot of pointing by Adalgesia to spot the asparagus spear. Skinny as a strand of wool and coloured camouflage-green, its stalk snaps beneath my fingers like a celebratory clap amid the morning birdsong. My frittata seems a lot of hard work away.

Happily Adalgesia's eyes are sharper than mine, and we already have more than enough to eat. With one hand she waves her asparagus harvest towards me and with the other gestures towards the sun. '*A casa!*' she decides. 'Home!' And she all but runs down the hill towards the stone farmhouse where she serves up four-course lunches daily for her husband.

Wild asparagus frittata is a signature springtime dish in Campo-dimele, and the first one villagers start talking about once word gets round that the season has started – that and the reminder that this plant is valued locally for its diuretic qualities, and will lend a grassy scent to your urine.

Frittata, the Italian alternative to the French omelette, takes only minutes to cook. It's delicious hot or cold so it's a versatile dish, good to eat instantly at home or slipped cold into picnic baskets. The Campomelani often eat it as a lunchtime *secondo*, perhaps with a *contorno* of oil-preserved peppers and aubergines, whose sweetness offers a contrast to the bitter asparagus. At special dinners frittata might appear as one of the antipasti.

Today Adalgesia is making me frittata for breakfast. Despite the hard work it has taken to source these spears, they are not afforded the delicate handling I've always understood the shop-bought stuff to require – the slow steaming in tall pans designed to protect the tips, the oil-bathed roasting. The wild spears are cleaned under fast-running cold water, rattled around a colander, then dumped onto the PVC kitchen tablecloth. Holding the root end of a spear in her left hand, Adalgesia snaps off the tip with her right hand then continues down the stem, snapping away 2 centimetre long pieces of green until her fingers feel the resistance of the woody lower stem, which she discards. Then she sploshes extra-virgin olive oil into the 25 centimetre non-stick pan she reserves for frittatas, heats the oil and flings in the asparagus pieces so that they fry over a high flame for a couple of minutes. Their taste is so strong, she responds to my quizzical eyebrow, that they can take the intense heat.

When you've worked this hard to find the filling for your frittata, only the finest eggs will do, and Adalgesia smiles as she cracks ten eggs of different sizes and various shades of brown into a glass bowl.

'*Caserecce*,' she nods approvingly towards the ones I've brought. *Caserecce*, 'home-produced', a classic tenet of the traditional Campodimele kitchen, and the highest accolade any food can be given round these parts. I found these ten eggs in a *macelleria*, a small independent butcher, in the nearby town of Lenola yesterday, and although their shells looked suitably rough, I had to wonder if a *contadina* had truly brought them direct from the hen house and her free-range, corn-fed birds, or if they would turn out to have been commercially produced. But you can tell these are *caserecce*, says Adalgesia, because of the freshness of their structure – the yolks stand tall, round as a full moon, vibrant as a sinking sun, and rest on a high bed of albumen, which gives way to a wider pool of transparent white. These eggs are just a day or so old, and only *caserecce* eggs can get from hen to kitchen that fast. 'No chemicals,' she adds. 'Like the asparagus.'

She flings in a handful of chopped flat-leaf parsley which she snapped in passing from her herb garden on the way into the kitchen then places a wooden chair beside the stove and springs up onto it so that she can search in an overhead cupboard. I wince as she balances on the collapsible A-frame chair, her seventy-three-year-old legs just centimetres from the frying-pan handle and the bubbling oil.

'*Sale*,' she says, holding up a jar of salt. '*Non zucchero!*' she adds, pointing to the sugar canister on the shelf. 'Once I put sugar in the frittata by mistake! What a waste of wild asparagus!'

Eggs, parsley, salt in the bowl, she whisks the mixture to a bubbly froth with a metal fork then pours the yellow river into the frying pan so that it hisses and spits. Slowly she works a wooden spoon round the circumference of the pan, drawing the cooked edges of the frittata towards the centre so that the liquid gold that remains raw flows into the space created at the edges then heats and solidifies. Her Teflon pan is a modern tool that seems at odds with the traditional simplicity of her kitchen – the stone-flagged floor, the open fireplace. I'd expected a steel skillet seasoned to a natural non-stick finish over the course of a thousand rustic meals – the pan of a down-shifter's dreams. But Adalgesia looks puzzled when I ask her why she chooses non-stick. '*Non si attacca*,' she explains kindly, 'so it doesn't stick.'

After five minutes of manoeuvring the eggs, she covers the pan with a blue-and-white-patterned plate, flips the whole lot upside down and removes the pan to reveal the frittata, cooked side up. She slips it back into the pan, uncooked side down and, thirty seconds later, *è pronta*! Breakfast is served. The frittata's crust is like golden layers of crispy lace, its centre a parsley-perfumed creaminess punctuated by the grassy crunch of asparagus pieces. So this is what all the fuss is about.

This breakfast took just minutes to cook, but more than an hour to collect – with a small-holding to run, hens, goats and sheep to tend, and a vegetable garden a kilometre's walk down the road, asparagus frittata will surely be a rare treat for Adalgesia and her family?

She shakes her head. 'I'll be picking it throughout the season – and we'll be eating it throughout the year,' she says, and I realize she is snapping the remaining asparagus pieces into small sections and dividing them between polythene freezer bags. *Frozen* wild asparagus?

'Why not?' she responds. 'Put them in the frying pan straight from the freezer and they are almost as good as freshly picked.'

It's months later that I understand that these little segments of wild asparagus embody the purist but practical philosophy of the Campodimele kitchen: that a bit of organization today means you can enjoy the rewards of your hard work all year round; that preserved food is fine, so long as it doesn't involve chemical preservatives; that we can hold on to the best of the old ways while embracing the best of the new. The understanding that between past, present and future, a balance can be found.

Frittata di asparagi selvatici – Wild asparagus frittata

If wild asparagus spears are unavailable, use the youngest, freshest green asparagus you can find. All these recipes use short pieces of asparagus. To prepare these, hold the tip of the asparagus in one hand and the root end in the other. Snap off the tip and continue snapping down the stem until you feel the resistance of the woody stem, which should be discarded.

A non-stick pan – either Teflon-coated or home-seasoned to a non-stick finish – is essential for this recipe.

Twenty wild asparagus spears
Three splashes of extra-virgin olive oil
Ten fresh organic eggs
Fine sea salt
Handful of fresh flat-leaf parsley, finely chopped

Wash the asparagus spears in cold water, drain them, and snap them into pieces 2cm (1in) long, as described above.

Heat the olive oil in a 25cm (10in) non-stick frying pan over a moderately high flame, throw in the asparagus, and fry for two minutes, stirring occasionally with a wooden spatula.

Meanwhile crack the eggs into a large bowl along with two or three pinches of salt, to taste, and the flat-leaf parsley. Beat vigorously with a hand-whisk, trying to get as much air as possible into the mixture.

Once the asparagus tips have been frying for around two minutes, and before they brown, pour the eggs into the pan. Use the spatula to gently move the egg mixture around the pan, so the uncooked egg falls to the base while the cooked egg rises above them. Continue this for around four minutes, or until there remains just a thin layer of uncooked egg on the top of the frittata.

At this point use the spatula to tip up the edge of the frittata – if it's golden and crispy underneath, it's ready to be flipped; if not, allow it to fry a little longer.

When the base of the frittata is golden and crispy, remove the pan from the heat and place a flat pan lid or upside-down plate over the pan. Hold the pan handle with one hand, place the palm of your other hand over the pan lid or plate, and quickly flip the pan over so that the frittata is now cooked side up on the plate.

Return the empty pan to the heat, and gently slide the frittata back into the pan so that the uncooked egg is now on the bottom. Allow the frittata to cook for about thirty to sixty seconds more until the bottom is golden then quickly slide the frittata onto a plate.

Using a sharp knife, make three cuts north–south and three cuts east–west so the frittata is cut into squares. Eat hot or at room temperature.

Serves four to six.

Spaghetti con asparagi al sugo rosso —
Spaghetti with asparagus and red sauce

Use a large, deep pan to make the sauce so you can fling the spaghetti into it once cooked, to ensure every strand is bathed in the *sugo*.

Two or three splashes of extra-virgin olive oil
Twenty asparagus spears, snapped into short pieces (see page 84)
One medium-sized yellow onion, finely chopped
Splash of good dry white wine
750ml (1½ pints) conserved tomato sauce (see page 263)
Half a stick of freshest celery and leaves, lightly crushed
Large stalk of flat-leaf parsley
Fine sea salt
400g (14oz) dried spaghetti
Handful of chopped flat-leaf parsley to garnish (optional)

Heat the oil in a deep pan over a moderately high heat then throw in the asparagus and onion, and fry for a few minutes until the vegetables are softened, but not coloured.

Add a large splash of white wine to the pan, and allow to reduce a little.

Now add the tomato sauce, along with a small glass of cold water, the celery, the parsley and a good pinch of salt.

Bring the sauce to a slow boil then turn down the heat and simmer for around twenty minutes, stirring occasionally to prevent the sauce from sticking. By now much of the water should have evaporated, leaving behind a thick sauce. Reduce the heat to a slow bubble.

Now put the spaghetti on to cook – bring a large pan of salted water to the boil, and cook according to the instructions on the packet, usually around eight to ten minutes.

Once the spaghetti is cooked al dente, remove both pans from the heat. Drain the spaghetti through a colander, and tip it into the pan of tomato sauce. Stir carefully to ensure the sauce is well distributed among the pasta.

Serve the spaghetti in warmed bowls, sprinkled with chopped flat-leaf parsley, if desired.

Serves four.

Spaghetti con asparagi selvatici al sugo bianco — Spaghetti with wild asparagus in white sauce

A glass of good dry white wine is the perfect accompaniment to this simplest of sauces.

Four splashes of extra-virgin olive oil
Twenty wild asparagus spears, snapped into short pieces (see page 84)
One medium-sized yellow onion, finely chopped
Handful of fresh flat-leaf parsley, roughly chopped
Fine sea salt
400g (14oz) dried spaghetti

Heat the oil in a deep pan, and, once it is hot, throw in the asparagus pieces, onion, parsley and a pinch or two of salt, and fry over a moderately high flame for around ten minutes – do not allow the vegetables to brown.

While the sauce is cooking, boil a pan of salted water, and cook the pasta according to the instructions on the packet, usually about eight to ten minutes.

Once the sauce and the pasta are cooked, remove both pans from the heat, drain the spaghetti and fling it into the pan of sauce. Stir gently to ensure each strand of pasta is coated with the sauce, and serve in warmed bowls.

Serves four.

April

The First Sign of Spring

Spring is here. You catch it in the watery smile of the morning sun, the unexpected warmth of the evening breeze, the star-studded clarity of the night sky. It floats in the air as apple-blossom white, blushes on the forest floor in smiles of cyclamen pink, sprouts out of the dark brown earth as the verdant shoots of shallots.

And it announces itself on the table as tumbling piles of little green broad beans, the food Italians traditionally regard as Nature's official first herald of *primavera*, spring. Not because they are the only beans available just now – the flat green *coralli*, which can be eaten entire with their pods, are here too, and the skinny, stringy *fagiolini*. But it's the broad beans with their wantonly curvaceous coats and their vivid green flesh which say most extravagantly that the dullness of winter is ended, the vibrancy of spring begun.

My neighbour Maria has been sitting on the stone wall beneath her walnut tree all day. It's the first time this year I've noticed her occupying this spot, her back to the new sun, and she's preparing broad beans. She snaps a pod in half, prises the four or five beans from the furry interior and discards the empty shell before starting over again with another pod.

The pile of pods is huge – I reckon 10 kilos or more. But the yield from each one is tiny, less than half their weight. Eagerly anticipated as broad beans are, they are a rude reminder that the laborious work of the land has returned along with the spring.

Maria invites me into her kitchen to prepare the beans. The room is a perfect mix of old and new, traditional and modern, a kitchen for people who love cooking and eating and who celebrate daily the goodness of food they produce with their own hands.

It's an L-shaped room with one leg devoted to the kitchen workspace – cream-coloured units and a stainless-steel hob: practical, attractive, modern, with none of the rustic nostalgia to which ex-pats in rural climes can be prone. But amid this oasis of mod cons are elements of the old days which still earn their place in the kitchen today – an open fireplace on which meat is grilled, and a *forno a legna* in which Maria bakes bread made from the wheat her husband, Michele, grows.

The corner angle is given over to seating, arranged around a television, and the second leg of the kitchen is swamped by a huge refectory table topped with a lemon-patterned PVC-coated cloth – the practical wipe-clean tablecloth found in every home here. Every Sunday a total of thirteen members of Maria's extended family gather for lunch around this table, and almost every mouthful they eat – meat, vegetables, fruit, wine, olives, bread – is produced by Maria and Michele on their *terreno*.

Tonight Maria and Michele will be eating *fave in umido* – broad beans stewed with onions and tomatoes. In days gone by, when money was scarce, families larger and meat a rare luxury, *fave in umido* was one of many bean dishes served as a *secondo*. Like *coralli in umido* and *fagiolini*, they offered a dish rich in protein and carbohydrates, but low in fat, nutritious and satisfying food to come home to after a morning working the land.

Today Maria still cooks broad beans *in umido*, but like most people she serves them as a *contorno*.

After Maria's long morning podding beans beneath the branches of her walnut tree, the preparation of the dish takes just minutes – a splash of olive oil in a deep pan, a chopped onion fried for a minute or two, a celery stick. Then in with the beans, half a bottle of home-made tomato sauce and a little water. A lid on the pan and after thirty minutes over a moderate flame the beans are stewed, little packets of earthy sweetness exploding from their wrinkled skins. The small, younger beans can be cooked along with their skins, explains Maria, but the skins of the bigger, older beans can be bitter and should be removed before cooking.

Today, however, we are shelling even the youngest, tiniest beans to make the dish with which the first broad beans are traditionally celebrated: *insalata di fave e pecorino* – broad bean and pecorino cheese salad. This dish is synonymous with spring in Rome and throughout the Lazio region. At this time of year it can be found on every menu, often served as an antipasto accompaniment to a pre-lunch glass of sparkling *prosecco*. Often you have to slip the beans out of their skins yourself at the table, but Maria prefers to do this for her guests. She makes a little mountain of skinned broad beans on a plate, surrounds them with thin slices of matured pecorino, a hard sheep's cheese, drizzles the beans with extra-virgin olive oil then sprinkles them with powdered *peperoncino*. This last addition is not a typical accompaniment to spring broad beans throughout the region, but *peperoncino* is the omnipresent condiment in Campodimele, and Maria sprinkles it over every meal, convinced it's as health-giving as it is delicious.

The combination of flavours is complex and explosive – the sweet mustiness of the beans, the saltiness of the cheese, the fruitiness of the oil, the fieriness of the chillies. A chunk of Maria's bread, tinged with the smokiness of her wood oven, and this is a main course in itself. A glass of Michele's home-made red wine, and this simple salad is a feast. Apart from the cheese, everything on the plate was home-produced. What products does Maria buy? '*Sale*,' she says. '*E zucchero. Pesce*' – fish. She shrugs. That's pretty much it. I sense that if she could produce these items at home, then she would.

The next day as I take my morning espresso onto my verandah to catch the heat of the sun spilling down the mountains, I find Maria again sitting under her walnut tree, working away at what looks like another pile of beans. And the next day, and the one after that. '*In campagna, c'è sempre da fare!*' she tells me. In the countryside, there is always something to do. This is just the start of such jobs, she adds; in the summer it never stops, I'll be seeing her out here a lot. And I realize that in Campodimele it is not just the broad beans that announce that winter is over; that here, beneath her walnut tree, Maria too is a symbol of spring.

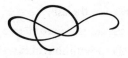

Fave in umido — Broad bean stew

1kg (2lb 3oz) young broad beans in their pods
Good splash of extra-virgin olive oil
One medium-sized golden onion, chopped
One stick of celery, crushed
500ml (1 pint) conserved tomato sauce (see page 263)
Fine sea salt

First shell the broad beans, and, if they are big, pop them out of their bitter skins.

Heat the oil in a deep pan, and fry the onion and celery stick for a few minutes until the onion is translucent, but not coloured.

Add the shelled beans and stir well before adding the tomato sauce and a small glass of cold water.

Bring gently to the boil, cover the pan with a lid, and simmer gently for around thirty to forty minutes, until the beans are tender.

Add salt to taste about ten minutes before the beans have finished cooking.

To make *fave in umido* out of season using dried broad beans, first soak 300g (11oz) dried weight of beans overnight in cold water, rinse well, and simmer gently for forty-five minutes to an hour until the beans have softened, but still retain plenty of bite. Then add them to the pan after the onion has fried gently, and simmer along with the other ingredients for around thirty minutes, adding the salt at the very end.

Serves four.

Coralli in umido – Stewed helda beans

Coralli is a dialectical name the Campomelani and the fruit and vegetable vendors of Fondi and the surrounding towns give to flat, green, stringless helda beans.

500g (1lb 2oz) coralli beans
Good splash of extra-virgin olive oil
One medium-sized golden onion, chopped
One clove of fresh garlic, thinly sliced
500ml (1 pint) conserved tomato sauce (see page 263)
Fine sea salt

Top and tail the beans, and cut into two halves down the middle.

Heat the oil in a deep pan and fry the onion for a few minutes until it is translucent, but not coloured.

Add the garlic and cook gently for a minute further.

Add the beans and stir well then add the tomato sauce, a glass of cold water and a good pinch of salt. Bring to the boil, cover and simmer for around thirty minutes, or until the beans are tender.

Add two or three good pinches of salt, to taste.

Serves four to six as a side dish.

Fagiolini con pomodoro, cipolla e prezzemolo — Green beans with tomato, onion and parsley

1 kg (2lb 3oz) green beans
Good splash of extra-virgin olive oil
One medium-sized golden onion, finely chopped
Good handful of fresh flat-leaf parsley, finely chopped
Fine sea salt
500ml (1 pint) conserved tomato sauce (see page 263) or six
   fresh, ripe plum tomatoes, skinned, deseeded and roughly
   chopped

Top and tail the beans, and boil in a large pan of salted water for about twenty minutes, less if you prefer your beans to have plenty of crunch.

While the beans are cooking, heat the oil in a deep pan and gently fry the onion until it is translucent.

Add the parsley, and fry for thirty seconds more then add salt to taste along with the tomato sauce and bring the sauce to a gentle simmer.

When the beans are ready, drain them then tip them into the pan of sauce, mix well, and serve hot or cold.

Serves four to six.

Carciofini for the Cantina

Can any place evoke a sense of peace and plenty as immediately as an Italian country *cantina*? I can't imagine so.

These cool, dark larders whisper of plans imagined and realized. Their shelves record the riches of harvests new in, and foretell the tale of the table in the year to come.

I can still remember the first time I stepped into Leana's Campodimele *cantina*, never guessing at the wealth I'd find behind the simple wooden door that shields it from the cobbled lane. The shaft of sunlight that slipped in behind me sparkled on twelve months of Nature preserved: the pork sausage Leana air-dries every January and keeps in jars of olive oil; the bottles of tomato sauce she conserves in summer; autumn fruits turned into sugary jam; green winter vegetables preserved in vinegar and oil. I caught the scent of onions garlanded and hung to dry, scanned the shadowy forms of demijohns filled with home-made red wine and olive oil.

When do you start this exaggerated store-cupboard, I wanted to ask. What's the season to begin?

The thought barely there, the answer was obvious: you start now. Because preserving the fruits of the *orto* is a never-ending cycle here.

And now, with winter gone, preserving routines move up several gears. One of the first crops to preserve are *carciofini*, baby globe artichokes. And so I'm in the kitchen with 'Pina and pile upon pile of *carciofini*. They are beautiful – little sculptural globes of overlapping leaves, their matt-green foliage streaked with violet which bleeds onto your hands as you hack your way to the golden hearts.

The staining power of artichokes is just one factor which prompted my long-held aversion to preparing them. The mere mention of this aristocrat of the thistle family is enough to make my fingertips prickle with the memory of the spiky tendrils of the choke that guards the edible heart.

Catherine de' Medici was said to have had a passion for artichokes and she is credited with having imported them to her adopted homeland of France in the sixteenth century – but I doubt that the woman who became the consort of Henry II of France ever had to prepare them herself.

Then again, artichokes are different here. *Carciofi*, the full-grown artichokes that arrive in November and are just available still, have no spikes, barely even a downy crown upon the heart. And *carciofini* still are too young to have developed the choke – they are all tender heart, wrapped in silky leaves, perfect for preserving in oil and storing in dark *cantine* until you want to eat them.

'Pina's kitchen is almost a thousand years old, part of a stone house accessed by a stone stairwell in the *centro storico*. Today the kitchen is dressed with what I will come to recognize as the familiar tools of *la conservazione* in Campodimele: bottles of white-wine vinegar, extra-virgin olive oil and a pot of salt, used for both its flavouring and its preservative powers. Then there are the condiments: *peperoncino*; the equally ubiquitous fresh flat-leaf parsley; slices of garlic, fresh from the fields just now and dried in clusters for use all year.

On the Formica table there is a range of sterilized glass jars with screw tops. The jars have been used before and still bear their old commercial labels: *melanzane arrostite*, declares one – roasted aubergines; another advertises *piselli* – garden peas – by Valfrutta, the brand of preserved foods that can be found on shop shelves throughout Italy.

The recycled jars bring to mind the re-used plastic mineral-water bottles full of dried pulses that I've spotted in *cantine* and the Coca-Cola bottles into which I've seen extra-virgin olive oil decanted from huge stainless-steel drums for transportation to the kitchen.

Storage here is about practicality, effectiveness, the quality of the food within, the workmanship that went into it. The aesthetic value is neither here nor there – all that matters is that the jars have been scrupulously sterilized, and that they will do the job that they are intended to do. I could blush when I think of the time I spent selecting shop-bought glass jars to store my home-made jam and marmalade back in the UK, so they would sit prettily on my kitchen shelves. 'We conserve everything!' 'Pina says, indicating her jars and expressing the local philosophy of *non buttiamo via niente*. We don't throw anything away.

Artichokes have never been so appealing, I think as I watch her snap on rubber gloves to protect her from the dye and set to work with a sharp knife: a swift horizontal swipe to remove the stem and base, a second horizontal slash to cut away the tops of the leaves. Loosened by these incisions, the tougher outer leaves scatter like confetti, leaving the tender and edible inner leaves hugging the heart. She drops it into a bowl of water laced with lemon juice, *acqua acidulata*, which will stop the hearts discolouring, and begins the process again.

As 'Pina works, a pan of white-wine vinegar diluted with water bubbles on the stove, and when she has a couple of dozen artichoke hearts ready, she drops them into the pan to simmer for a few minutes – just long enough to soften a little and take on the taste of the vinegar. She tips the *carciofini* into a colander to drain, and the vinegar water bubbles out of the leaves so that they look like yellow rosebuds drenched with dew.

Drying *carciofini* is of paramount importance before putting them *sott'olio*, says 'Pina in her Italian-accented English. 'Pina's parents moved from Campodimele to England in the lean years after the war, and she was born in Oxfordshire, returning with them to their native village when she was fourteen. She became my first friend in Campodimele when she astonished me by welcoming me to her bar on the piazza in English, saying, 'We are all looking forward to helping you.' She's been helping me endlessly ever since. 'As my father says,' 'Pina tells me now, 'preserved foods are like a house – if water gets inside when you make the foundations, it falls down.'

To dry thoroughly, the *carciofini* must be turned upside down on a clean tea towel and left there for twelve hours at least – perhaps longer – if they are to remain good for up to a year. But we are going to eat this batch over the next few days, so the drying is not so important. 'Pina dries a dozen or so with a tea towel, slices them in half and mixes them in a bowl with extra-virgin olive oil and *condimenti*: a little chilli pepper, a few sprigs of parsley, a clove of sliced, fresh garlic and some finely ground sea salt. She adds some fresh oregano and dried mint.

She then piles the *carciofini* into a glass jar and carefully fills it with olive oil, tilting the jar to ensure all the artichokes are covered and that no air bubbles remain. Then she seals it with a screw-top lid and hands it to me. These will keep well in the fridge for a few days, by which time the flavours will have had a chance to meld and mature.

But they don't last that long. The very next day, I open the jar to nibble the *carciofini* as antipasti before lunch and find myself unable to stop eating them – the creamy smoothness of the hearts is cut by the sharp tang of vinegar, the hot sparks of chilli at war with the cool notes of the mint. I wipe the flavoured oil out of the jar with chunks of bread. I want more of these artichokes. I want to eat them all year round. I want a *cantina* packed with them.

I don't have an *orto* yet, because I don't have a garden, and I don't have a *cantina* to call my own. But that doesn't matter, because a *cantina* is not just a place – it's a mentality, a system of food, a way of life. I realize you can create a *cantina* anywhere, if you have a mind to, and not just with home-grown crops, but with produce which is bought.

And so my *cantina* in Campodimele starts with carrier bags full of *carciofini* bought from the *frutta verdura*, the huge fruit-and-veg van which Anna and Franco navigate up the winding mountain road from Fondi twice a week, selling fresh produce to those who do not grow their own. I do this within the week, because if I wait longer than that, the *carciofini* season will be gone. I empty a kitchen cupboard of dishes, wipe the shelves down then arrange my jars of *carciofini* in neat rows.

It's hardly the *cantina* of my dreams. It's not a stone-walled room behind a rickety wooden door into which I can step to see and scent and stroke my fingers along a year's worth of my own home-grown food. But this is a start. These sixteen jars of *carciofini* foretell something of what I will eat during the year to come. Four jars I'll give to friends, when I visit for dinner or when they drop by, because exchanging your home preserves is part of life's everyday loveliness here. A dozen I'll keep for myself, reaching into my *cantina* to draw down a jar once a month, to serve as antipasti, as a *contorno* or as an instant way of padding out a meal when unexpected guests arrive – the fast food, slow style mentality of what I think of as *cantina cucina*. In the summer I will do the same with aubergines, and in September with hot chillies and sweet peppers too. In autumn I'll turn apricots into jam to last me through the winter. And so here, in my Formica-fronted wall-cupboard, the one next to the kitchen window, where the contents will stay cool, I find my sense of peace and plenty: the satisfaction of the moment seized, the year ahead secured.

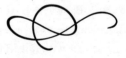

Insalata di carciofini – Baby artichoke salad

The artichokes most readily available outside Italy tend to have a spiky choke above the soft heart, and this needs to be removed before cooking. Baby artichokes are picked before the choke develops, so once you have removed the stem and outer leaves they can be eaten – cooked or raw.

If your artichoke leaves are purple, wear gloves to protect your hands.

This little salad may seem like a lot of work – but the results make the time spent worth it.

Twelve baby artichokes or nine large artichokes
One lemon
Fine sea salt
Extra-virgin olive oil
Handful of fresh flat-leaf parsley, chopped (optional)
Crushed dried red chilli (optional)

To prepare the artichokes, cut the stem away at the base of the bulb, and peel away the loosened outer leaves, which are too tough to eat.

Use a small spoon to scoop out the spiky chokes which lie above the heart, if using large artichokes.

Place the cut artichokes immediately into a bowl of water laced with the juice of half a lemon, to stop discolouring.

Slice the hearts thinly, from top to bottom, and place on a shallow serving dish.

Sprinkle them with salt, drizzle with the extra-virgin olive oil then squeeze the juice from the remaining half of the lemon over the raw artichokes and stir gently, ensuring each slice is coated with dressing – this is important to prevent discolouring.

Sprinkle with chopped parsley and a few pinches of chilli pepper, if using, and allow to rest for at least fifteen minutes before serving at room temperature.

Serves two to four as a side dish.

Carciofini sott'olio – Baby artichokes preserved in oil

Baby artichokes can be hard to come by outside the Mediterranean, but older ones are also good to preserve in oil – just be sure to remove every last layer of tough leaves, the tough stalk at the base and the thorny choke. The amounts of artichokes and oil you need will depend on the size of the artichokes and the size of the jars you are using. Fifteen baby artichokes for a 500 millilitre (1 pint) jar is a rough guide – the amount below is enough for two such jars. Hygiene is paramount when preserving food in oil, so be sure to sterilize the jars thoroughly (see page 188).

Thirty baby artichokes or twenty large artichokes
1 litre (2 pints) white-wine vinegar
Around 500ml (1 pint) extra-virgin olive oil, possibly more
Crushed dried red chilli
Two cloves of fresh garlic, finely sliced
Few pinches of dried mint
Few pinches of dried oregano
Fine sea salt
Few fresh flat-leaf parsley sprigs
Two 500ml (1 pint) glass jars with screw tops, sterilized

Prepare the artichokes according to the instructions on page 104.

Boil the white-wine vinegar in a large pan together with 1 litre (2 pints) of water.

Add the artichoke hearts, return the pan to the boil, and simmer for three to four minutes, but no longer.

Drain the artichoke hearts into a colander and shake well.

When the artichoke hearts are cool enough to handle, dry them gently with a clean tea towel or kitchen paper. Place a clean tea towel on a flat surface in a cool place, and arrange the hearts upside down so any excess water can drain out. They should be left like this for at least twelve hours or even overnight – change the tea towel if it becomes too damp to allow effective drying.

When the artichokes are dry enough to bottle, sterilize the glass jars (see page 188).

Place the dry artichokes in a large bowl, add a splash or two of extra-virgin olive oil, then add the dried chilli, sliced garlic, dried mint and oregano, and a sprinkling of fine sea salt – a couple of good pinches of each herb and spice should suit most tastes, or add more or less if you prefer. Add the parsley sprigs. Mix thoroughly to ensure each heart comes into contact with all of the flavourings.

Pour a small splash of olive oil into the bottom of each of the sterilized jars, then spoon in the artichokes, leaving around 2cm (1in) of space at the tops of the jars. Pour olive oil into the jars, tilting them from side to side as you go to ensure all the artichokes are coated and to encourage any air bubbles to rise to the top. Make sure the artichokes are completely covered with oil before screwing tight-fitting lids into place.

The artichokes can be eaten instantly, but will taste better if the flavours are allowed to meld over a few weeks. Store in a cool, dark place. Once opened, store in the fridge and eat within a day or two.

Makes two 500ml (1 pint) jars.

Carciofi in umido con aglio, prezzemolo, peperoncino e scarola
— Artichokes stewed with garlic, parsley, chilli pepper
and scarola lettuce

Scarola is a kind of spiky-leafed lettuce which can be eaten raw as a salad, but here is commonly eaten cooked, with a little salt and olive oil, or added to *minestre*, the thick vegetable soups that make a delicious first course in winter or summer. Wilted *scarola* tastes delicious with artichokes, but this dish works just as well without it.

Juice of half a lemon
Twelve large artichokes
Few splashes of extra-virgin olive oil
Two cloves of garlic, finely chopped
Handful of fresh flat-leaf parsley, finely chopped
Good pinch of crushed dried red chilli
Fine sea salt
Half a scarola lettuce, leaves separated and washed

Squeeze the lemon juice into a bowl of cold water in order to create acidulated water to stop the peeled artichokes discolouring.

Prepare the artichokes according to the instructions on page 104, and steep in the acidulated water until ready.

In a small bowl, mix the extra-virgin olive oil with the chopped garlic, chopped parsley, crushed chilli and a pinch or two of salt.

One by one, remove the artichokes from the acidulated water and dry on a clean tea towel then spoon a little of the olive-oil mixture over each one, ensuring plenty of the oil reaches the heart and slithers between the layers of leaves.

Splash a little olive oil over the base of a large, shallow pan, and arrange the artichokes upside down in the pan. Add a glass of cold water.

Place the *scarola* leaves over the upturned artichokes, drizzle over a very little oil and a sprinkling of salt, then cover the pan with a lid. Heat gently until you can hear the water starting to simmer, then lower the heat and stew for around half an hour, or until the artichoke hearts are tender to the point of a sharp knife. Check occasionally to ensure there is still a little water in the base of the pan, adding just a little more should it all evaporate.

This is best served hot as a side dish.

Serves four to six.

Carciofi in umido con mentuccia, aglio e prezzemolo –
Artichokes stewed with mint, garlic and parsley

Juice of half a lemon
Twelve large artichokes
Few splashes of extra-virgin olive oil
Small handful of fresh, chopped mint leaves or good pinch of dried
*   mint*
Two cloves of garlic, finely chopped
Handful of fresh flat-leaf parsley, finely chopped
Fine sea salt
Half a scarola lettuce, leaves separated and washed

Follow the recipe on page 108 to prepare the artichokes, but instead of adding dried chilli to the olive-oil dressing, add a small handful of chopped fresh mint.

Serves four to six.

Morning on the Mountain

Goat bells are the music to which Campodimele slides into sleep and stirs. By day you catch their occasional note as the wind sweeps up to the village from the shepherds' settlement of Pozzo della Valle. Or a concentrated clanging as the goatherds guide their animals to fresh grazing grounds. As dusk falls and the background buzz of the day subsides, the goat bells become the slow song of the evening, fading with the night, only floating on the air again as the cockerel crows.

That's how it is today, on the hillside, as Adamo gathers his goats. It's 6.30 a.m. and the sun is slipping over the mountain peaks to dance with the mist, as if lured by the tune of the bells. In a wooden-fenced enclosure, beneath a canopy of oak trees, the goats skitter with the excitement of the new day. Mothers bleat answers to the cries of their kids, young males lock hornless heads in momentary fights, shaggy white dogs with silly faces bark and yelp.

Amid this quiet commotion Adamo commences *la mungitura*, the twice-daily ritual of milking the goats. He strides between the animals and, one by one, grasps their hind legs, places a metal pail beneath their udders and squats to squeeze the milk from their teats.

There's something timeless about this scene: the mountains, unspoiled throughout millennia, the goats, an ancient symbol of Nature or the Devil, depending on which culture you adhere to. Adamo himself could be from another age, I think, with his huge moustache and the leather ties of his *cioce* criss-crossing up his shins. Until I see that these shepherd's shoes are, like so many things around here, a perfect marrying of the modern and the old – tops of handcrafted goatskin, soles created from old car tyres, their treads ideal for the mountainous terrain.

La mungitura finished, Adamo disappears into his tin hut, emerging with a tray of tiny cups brimming with espresso.

'*Cento animali*,' he says, indicating his herd. A hundred goats to be milked first thing in the morning and last thing at night, from Easter to mid-September. About 100 litres of milk a day in good weather, 50 daily when autumn comes. In the summer, Adamo often sleeps here, passing the hours carving wooden collars for his goats, to which he attaches the brass bells whose chorus enchants the mountain. Twice a day he carts the milk the few kilometres down the mountain to his farmhouse in Taverna, where his wife, Evelina, transforms it into cheese. Which is where I head now.

'*Adamo ed Evelina!*' She smiles at the coincidence of hers and her husband's names. Adam and Eve. The first man and woman to walk the Earth, according to the Old Testament, and I can't help thinking that goatherds were working like this, and their womenfolk crafting cheese this way, when that biblical story was written down.

Evelina's kitchen is modern, but her cheese-making methods are ages old. This morning she is working on yesterday evening's batch of milk. Last night she doused it with *coagulo* – rennet scraped from the stomach of one of their baby goats, and this has done its job of coagulating the milk fats so they have separated from the watery whey.

Evelina makes the cheese with the help of her *mallia* – a large wooden tray balanced at a shallow angle on three wooden chairs – and *cestini*, cylindrical cheese moulds fashioned from plastic mesh. She fills one of the little moulds with the lumpy curds and, placing a hand on each end, tips it to and fro so that the whey trickles through the mesh. The milky liquid drains down the *mallia*, through an open lip at its lower end and into a waiting bucket. The more she agitates the curds, the more whey spills out, until she is left with a solid lump of *formaggio* – cheese.

Evelina invites me to copy her and hands me a *cestino* full of curds: they are snowy-white and dense, heavier than they look, and I enjoy feeling the cheese slowly form beneath my wet hands.

When the last of the curds have been turned into *formaggio*, Evelina rolls them in coarse-grained salt and sets them to rest for two days, during which time the salt will draw the moisture from the cheese, making it firm and ready to eat.

Later she will make ricotta, she says, lifting the bucket into which the whey has drained. *Ricotta* literally means 'recooked': Evelina heats the whey in a pan over a naked flame, and the fat remaining curdles and rises to the surface to be skimmed off and slipped into round, flat moulds. The ricotta will be eaten fresh, perhaps with a slick of olive oil and hot chilli pepper, as an accompaniment to bread. Or swirled into pasta. But the *formaggio* can be preserved, Evelina tells me, *sott'olio* or *sotto vuoto* – vacuum-packed in plastic for up to three years.

This modern method of preservation seems so at odds with Evelina's age-old method of making cheese, but is in fact no surprise to me now. I have understood that modern technology has a role to play in the creation of *cibo genuino*, so long as it doesn't adulterate the food with chemicals or in some other way. But even as Evelina is explaining how modern advances help her store her cheese for years, I can't help wondering how long this traditional way of cheese-making will survive.

'It's a good life,' says Maria Civita, Evelina's mother. She is over seventy, but can often be seen by the roadside in Taverna, watching silently over the family's flock of sheep. She's one of many shepherds still in these parts: sometimes you'll round a bend and find yourself in the middle of a four-legged traffic jam. Maria Civita became a shepherd when she was fourteen and still loves the fact that she works outdoors, that she is not confined to an indoor life.

'I don't even like wearing a coat with sleeves, whatever the weather,' she told me one day as we gazed at her sheep grazing in a field. 'I feel freer without them. Free outside.' But it's a tough life: working outdoors in all weathers, early mornings, late finishes, tied to the grazing ground and milking the animals, or to the farmstead, making cheese.

Up on his mountain top, rising with the sun, Adamo must feel free, with only Nature to tell him what to do. But such rural idylls require their sacrifices too, I think, as we head off to the village and leave him with only the sound of the goatbells to disturb his thoughts.

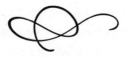

Frittata di ricotta – Ricotta omelette

You'll need a 25 centimetre (10 inch) wide frying pan with a non-stick finish for this.

Ten fresh organic eggs
Fine sea salt
200g (7oz) fresh goat's cheese ricotta
Good splash of extra-virgin olive oil

Break the eggs into a bowl and beat vigorously with a good pinch of salt. Add the ricotta to the eggs bit by bit, beating between additions.

Heat the oil in a large frying pan over a medium flame, and pour in the mixture. Heat the eggs for a minute or so then, using a wooden spatula, gently pull the egg mixture from the edges of the pan towards the centre. Tilt the pan so the liquid egg in the centre slides to the edges to cook.

Lift the edge of the omelette to check if the underside is lightly golden, and, when it is, place a flat plate on top of the frying pan. Holding the pan handle in one hand and the plate in the other, flip the pan so the omelette drops onto the plate. Place the pan back on the stove, slide the omelette back into the pan uncooked side down, and allow it to cook for a further minute or so, until the underside is golden.

Cut into squares and serve hot or cold.

Serves four to six.

Ricotta con olio e peperoncino –
Ricotta with olive oil and peperoncino

This is a delicious way to eat ricotta and a perfect snack or light lunch. Few people in Campodimele keep black pepper, but this works very well with that too, if you prefer.

400g (14oz) fresh ricotta
Small vessel of extra-virgin olive oil
Crushed dried red chilli
Lots of fresh, crusty bread

Place the ricotta on a serving plate, and allow diners to cut away a portion of the cheese, splash it with olive oil, sprinkle crushed chilli over it then eat it with lots of good crusty bread.

Serves four.

Spaghetti alla ricotta – Spaghetti with ricotta sauce

Deceptively delicious, this dish is simplicity itself.

400g (14oz) spaghetti
400g (14oz) fresh ricotta
Fine sea salt
Good splash of extra-virgin olive oil
Crushed dried red chilli

Bring a large pan of salted water to the boil, add the spaghetti, and cook according to the instructions on the packet.

While the pasta is cooking, gently place the ricotta in a large bowl with a pinch or two of salt and gently beat it to a creamy consistency.

When the spaghetti is cooked al dente, drain it, add it to the bowl of ricotta, and gently stir it, using two forks, to coat every strand of pasta.

Divide into warmed serving bowls, and sprinkle over some crushed chilli and a splash of extra-virgin olive oil, if desired. Serve immediately.

Serves four.

MAY

Salad Days

Pasqualina has travelled 7,000 kilometres to spend the summer in her native Campodimele, but barely has she arrived and she's raising salad greens.

There's the *cappuccio*, she tells me, with its round, squat, rose-like formation of leaves, and the *Romana*, with its long, slender ribbed sheafs of green. And another which Pasqualina can't identify just now. 'Just *insalata*,' she says. '*Buona*, whatever it's called. A lot of Italians keep an *orto* at home in Toronto, just like here. But the stuff we grow in Canada doesn't taste like this.'

Pasqualina and her late husband, Michele, were among the thousands of Campomelani who left Italy in the post-war years to seek opportunities abroad. They settled in Toronto, which today is home to around 3,500 people of Campomelano descent. After Michele retired, he and Pasqualina found time to spend their summers in Campodimele. The village lures its children back with its pure air, the restorative powers of the sun, the tranquil rhythms of pastoral life. The unforgettable food.

Pasqualina's *orto* has the air of a secret garden. From the cobbled street you slip through a wrought-iron gate, step down a stone staircase, then dip your head to squeeze through an archway cut low into the grapevine-wreathed fence. Inside you find a bed of courgettes rampant, salad tomatoes, rows of salad greens. Cast your gaze upwards and you meet the sweep of the mountains and acre upon acre of heaven-blue, gold-streaked sky. It feels like the top of the world, the only place in the world. How must it have felt to emigrate from here all those decades ago? To fly across the globe to a strange city, never knowing if you would make it back, if you would ever see the people you loved again?

Happily, most émigrés do make it back from time to time, and even when they are thousands of kilometres away, you only have to spend an hour or two in the village to realize that their presence is ever felt here. It seems everyone in Campodimele has a brother, a child, a cousin overseas. Elderly women recount tales of visits to Toronto and display snapshots set against the backdrop of Niagara Falls. Children talk excitedly of forthcoming holidays *con i cugini, e gli zii*, with their cousins and aunts and uncles, in America or London. In the centre of the village a huge multicoloured mosaic depicts the emigrant experience of Campodimele. Plainly dressed *contadini* represent the difficult life after the war, while richly dressed figures bearing musical instruments symbolize the life of plenty some of Campodimele's children found overseas.

Pasqualina says that back home in Toronto, many Campomelani recreate the *cucina* of the village they left behind, not just at the table, but in their larders full of preserves, in the *orti* of their back-yards – and who can blame them?

'People make fresh pasta with eggs, conserve bottles of tomato sauce, keep an *orto* – just like here.' And they grow salad greens, an essential part of every Italian meal.

Pasqualina snaps a head of *Romana* lettuce out of the ground, plucks some greeny-orange San Marzano tomatoes from the vine and takes me back to the kitchen of her stone house. Fresh and juicy, the lettuce feels heavy for its size, its spine stiff as a stick, its leaves crunchy crisp. The tomatoes explode with tartness, deliciously under-ripe. Pasqualina dresses the salad in the way they do it here – splashing extra-virgin olive oil, white-wine vinegar and fine sea salt straight onto the leaves. Something this simple can only taste delicious if the ingredients are exceptionally fresh, unquestionably good – and, grown just metres away from this kitchen, just minutes old, they are. Little wonder Campomelani maintain this tradition thousands of kilometres away across the globe. As best as they can, that is.

Pasqualina slices a bulb of fennel, rinses it under a tap and splashes the vegetable with balsamic vinegar, creating a salad with the speed and simplicity which only the most flavoursome fresh vegetables allow.

'It's just that in Toronto we don't have this sun,' she says, gesturing to the brightness that floods through her kitchen window from the cobbled piazza outside. 'The air and the soil there are different – maybe not so pure. *Bello il Canadà, sì,* but the food in our *orti* over there, it never tastes quite like this.'

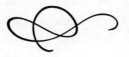

Insalata semplice – Simple salad

This is so simple that it can barely be described as a recipe
– the sort of plain, everyday green salad eaten here daily
after the *secondo*.

One Romana lettuce or another kind of green-leaf lettuce
Best extra-virgin olive oil
White-wine vinegar
Fine sea salt

At least fifteen minutes before you wish to eat the salad,
wash, shred and use a salad-spinner to dry the lettuce, then
place it in a large bowl.

Splash over some extra-virgin olive oil and a little white-
wine vinegar, and sprinkle over some salt.

Mix well using two forks, taste, and adjust the flavourings if necessary. Allow to rest to allow the flavourings to
penetrate.

Serves four to six.

Insalata mista al limone –
Mixed-leaf salad with fennel and lemon juice

One Romana lettuce
One red radicchio
One small bunch of rocket
One bulb of fennel
Extra-virgin olive oil
Fine sea salt
Juice of half a lemon

At least fifteen minutes before serving the salad, wash, shred and use a salad-spinner to dry the leaves, then place them in a large bowl.

Remove the tough outer leaves from the fennel, wash and finely shred the bulb, and add to the leaves.

Splash the salad with the olive oil, sprinkle with salt, and squeeze over the juice of half a lemon. Taste and adjust the condiments if necessary.

Serves four to six.

Insalata di pomodoro e cipolla – Tomato and onion salad

Handful of ripe, fresh plum tomatoes
Few spring onions or young golden onions
Extra-virgin olive oil
White-wine vinegar
Few pinches of fresh or dried oregano
Fine sea salt

Slice the tomatoes widthways and place in a bowl.

Strip the outer skin and green tails from the spring onions then slice the bulbs finely – or slice golden onions into the thinnest half-moons. Combine with the tomatoes.

Splash with extra-virgin olive oil and white-wine vinegar, and sprinkle over the fresh oregano and a little salt. If using dried oregano, make the salad at least half an hour before eating to allow the oil to penetrate and soften the dried herb.

Serves four to six.

Insalata di pomodoro, mozzarella e basilico –
Tomato, mozzarella and basil salad

Mozzarella di bufala, little white balls of fresh cheese made from buffalo milk, is traditional to the region of Campana, lying immediately to the south of Lazio. It is also produced in Itri, Lenola and Fondi, small towns which are a 30 minute drive down the mountain from the village. Improved transport links have helped make buffalo mozzarella a staple across Italy. This salad is also delicious without the cheese.

Handful of ripe, fresh plum tomatoes
Four balls of mozzarella di bufala
Extra-virgin olive oil
Handful of fresh basil leaves
Fine sea salt
Freshly ground black pepper (optional)

Slice the tomatoes widthways, slice the mozzarella, and arrange alternate rings of tomatoes and mozzarella on the plate.

Splash with the olive oil and tear the fresh basil over the salad. Add salt and black pepper, if desired (though most Campomelani wouldn't dream of using it!).

Serves four.

From the Hen House

'*Pipee, pipeeee, pipeeeeeeeee!*'

I can hear Maria calling long before I see her, catch a sense of the commotion before I can tell where it's coming from. It's just after 3.00 p.m. on a sunny day, and I'm stooping to catch the scent of some cerise-coloured cyclamen someone has placed at Campodimele's statue of San Padre Pio. The recently beatified monk is venerated throughout Italy for the stigmata he's believed to have suffered during his time on Earth. But the view he enjoys from the crossroads here, down the sweep of the Liri Valley, must be among the finest he enjoys anywhere. Then the noise begins.

There's no ignoring the din, because it's usually so quiet at this time of day just now. Lunch is over, the siesta hour is here, so the tractors and chainsaws are holding their tongues. The winter winds have become bored of their blowing, and there's barely the whisper of a breeze in the leafing trees. On these spring afternoons there's a sort of stillness which slows the heartbeat, soothes the soul so much that just here, just now, under this endless sky, you feel you really could live forever.

All of which makes the racket more noticeable. I follow my curious ears up the hill, to the sloping road that runs along the eastern flank of the village, and find myself beside the run of low stone outbuildings which line the road: *le galline*.

Le galline means many things in Campodimele. It literally translates as 'the hens', and at its simplest it refers to the birds many of the older ladies in particular keep for *uova caserecce*, home-produced eggs, and the occasional *brodo* made from boiled chicken and used as a basis for soups. *Le galline* is also a geographical term of reference for the road that skirts the back of the village – a road whose official name I have therefore never felt the need to learn. *Le galline* is also a time of day here – in temperate weather it means roughly 3.00 p.m., in the hottest months closer to 4.00 p.m., the time of day when the women rise from their siestas and go to put the free-range birds to bed for the night. '*Dopo le galline*', 'after the hens', is the most frequent phrase added to an invitation to pop round for coffee, late afternoon.

This is what all the fuss is about: Maria is trying to coax her hens into their house, but the russet-feathered birds will not cooperate. I can't see Maria to start with, but I can hear her: '*Pipeee! Pipeeeeee!*' Nobody can tell me what this word means, certainly not the dictionary. But it's the official call used by everyone here to bring the hens home. The shouts are coming from overhead, and, raking my gaze up a steep, soily bank, I spot Maria.

'*Vieni!*' she shouts, inviting me up to the *casettina*, the little house where her hens sleep, but as I step off the road my walking boots slither backwards on the shifting soil of the stony hillside, and I decide to stay put. Maria, who is wearing smooth-soled, brown slip-on house shoes, seems unbothered by the treacherous terrain. She has persuaded one of the hens into its house, but three others are dallying behind a tree at the top of the bank, casting her the odd dismissive glance as they forage for grubs. Who can blame them for wanting to stay outside on a day like today, with the sun still hot and dazzling? Maria doesn't agree. She stoops to grab a stick and throws it in the direction of the tree. When that fails to work, she stoops to grab a handful of stones, stomps up the bank and chucks the missiles one by one so that they land behind the birds. The hens are barely startled, but apparently admit collective defeat and, as one, strut slowly towards their den, pecking up the odd grub along the way.

The hen house is cool inside, with just a shaft of light entering via a slit in the roof. There's a tray of corn, a bucket of water, a basket filled with fresh straw for the birds to bed down. With a little exclamation Maria stoops and swipes something out of the straw and hands it to me. It's an egg, the only egg today, still warm – from the sun, or the hen who laid it, I don't know. I'm reluctant to accept it, because I know that eggs are still an important part of the diet round here, but Maria insists. 'Eat it tonight!' she says, '*Fresca, fresca!*' – fresh, with a little olive oil, a little salt.

Maria has four hens, one aged three years, the others just five months. Despite their reluctance to follow her home, they let her gather them into her arms with only a perfunctory protest before relaxing against her embrace.

'*Piccoline!*' sighs Maria, 'very small', and she explains that the three younger hens are not eating and so not laying. Maria is eighty-three, and even after decades of keeping hens, she doesn't understand why these are not thriving. She takes my hand and presses it against the bird's chest, a soft rush of warm air escaping the feathers and enveloping my fingers. I can feel a slight swelling, which Maria explains is the hen's stomach, but it should be bigger. '*Mangia, mangia!*' she coos like a mother to a child and, holding a handful of corn against the hen's beak, persuades her to take a grain or two.

Outside we can hear Maria's friends calling their hens home, the clang of old iron bedsteads being weighted against flimsy hen-house doors, the scrape of rocks being repositioned as anchors on the terracotta tile roofs – protection against hungry foxes and night winds. We go outside to perch on the wall and chat. *Le galline* is a key part of the social fabric of Campodimele. While the men gather on the piazza to smoke and play cards, their womenfolk pause here to discuss the events of the day, how their hens are laying – and, as always with Italians, what they will be eating for dinner.

My dinner will be this *casereccio* egg fried in extra-virgin olive oil and sprinkled with salt and *peperoncino*. The yolk will, I know, be as golden as the field of corn which fed these hens, the albumen firm and high in the centre. It will taste of . . . well, of the freshest egg, but there will be no chemical tang, no blandness, just the unmistakeable richness of *cibo genuino*.

I wonder what the hen who made my dinner is called, and Maria laughs out loud. 'A name, for a hen? Whoever would do that?' English people, I say, especially if they only have four to a hen house. 'They're animals!' Maria points out. 'We keep them for food. And if they stop laying . . .' She swipes her hand across her throat, with an unsentimental smile: '*Brodo!*'

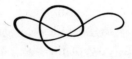

Pollo e patate – Chicken and potatoes

This is a quick and delicious one-pot oven roast. It's preferable to leave the skin on the chicken so that the fat bastes the vegetables, improving the whole taste of the dish. Some cooks here add chunks of red pepper too, but be sure to cut them large, to avoid them burning.

Slick of extra-virgin olive oil
600g (1 lb 5oz) potatoes suitable for oven-roasting, peeled
One medium-sized golden onion, thickly sliced
Handful of fresh flat-leaf parsley sprigs
Fine sea salt
Four garlic cloves, peeled and squashed by the side of a knife (optional)
Four fresh plum tomatoes, skinned and chopped (optional)
Two red peppers, quartered (optional)
One organic, free-range chicken jointed into eight pieces or a mixture of chicken pieces, with or without skin

Preheat the oven to 200°C/400°F/Gas Mark 6, and lightly grease a large roasting tin with just a slick of olive oil.

Cut the peeled potatoes into even-sized chunks, roughly 4cm (2in) square, and scatter over the bottom of the roasting tin.

Add the onion, parsley and a few good pinches of salt, along with the garlic, tomatoes and peppers, if using, and mix well with the potatoes.

Sprinkle salt over the chicken then place it in the tin, pressing it down into the vegetable and herb mix.

If you have left the skin on the chicken, drizzle just a little olive oil over it. If you have removed it, add a little more oil.

Place the roasting tin in the oven for around forty-five minutes to an hour – or until the chicken and potatoes are thoroughly cooked. Stir occasionally to ensure the flavours are well mixed, and baste the chicken in the pan juices. If the potatoes start to brown before the chicken is cooked through, place a piece of aluminium foil over the pan until everything is cooked.

Serves four to six.

Pollo alla brace – Chicken cooked over charcoal

Alla brace is still a typical way to cook meat in Campo-dimele, because most homes retain their open fires fuelled by wood – coal is not used. You can also use a barbecue or conventional grill for this recipe.

Four chicken pieces, preferably still attached to the skin and bone
Few splashes of extra-virgin olive oil
Pinch of fine sea salt
Few sprigs of fresh rosemary
Few cloves of garlic, peeled and squashed by the side of a knife

Place all the ingredients in a bowl, mix well, and allow to marinate in a cool place for at least an hour – or overnight in the fridge if possible.

If you are lucky enough to have a wood fire – or feel inclined to make one in your garden – slot the marinated chicken into a barbecue grid griller and place close to – but not on – the embers until the chicken is thoroughly cooked through. Or cook on a home barbecue.

Serves four.

Uova all'inferno – Eggs in hell

This dish gets its colourful name from the fact that it is traditionally cooked in a terracotta dish over the flames of the household's open fire. The smoke from the wood fire lends extra flavour to the eggs. Alternatively, cook them in a small frying pan over your cooker hob.

Splash of extra-virgin olive oil
Splash of conserved tomato sauce (see page 263) or two fresh plum tomatoes, skinned, deseeded and chopped
Two fresh organic eggs
Fine sea salt
Crushed dried red chilli

Place a slick of olive oil in a flame-proof terracotta dish then put a splash of tomato sauce or the chopped tomatoes on one side of the dish, and heat the tomatoes over the flames of your open fire or cooker.

When the tomatoes are heated through, crack the eggs onto the empty part of the dish and allow them to cook for two to three minutes, or until the tops of the yolks are milky-white.

Scatter with salt, to taste, and a little crushed chilli. Eat immediately, straight from the dish, along with lots of fresh, crusty bread.

Serves one.

Uova fritte con peperoncino –
Fried eggs with hot chilli pepper

It may seem ridiculous to include a recipe for fried eggs, but this dish sums up the unpretentiousness of the Campodimele *cucina* and the way it celebrates the very finest ingredients in the simplest of ways. This is regarded as the best way to fully enjoy the flavour of eggs which are *fresche, fresche*. The flavoursome quality of the olive oil is also paramount in a dish with so few ingredients.

Splash of extra-virgin olive oil
Two fresh organic eggs
Fine sea salt
Crushed dried red chilli

Heat the olive oil in a small frying pan and, when it is hot, crack the eggs into the pan, cover the pan with a lid, and lower the heat.

After two or three minutes, lift the lid – if the tops of the yolks are white and opaque, the eggs are probably cooked through, in which case remove the pan from the heat, sprinkle the eggs with salt and dried chilli, and eat them immediately – straight from the pan is best so they don't go cold – with lots of crusty bread.

Serves one.

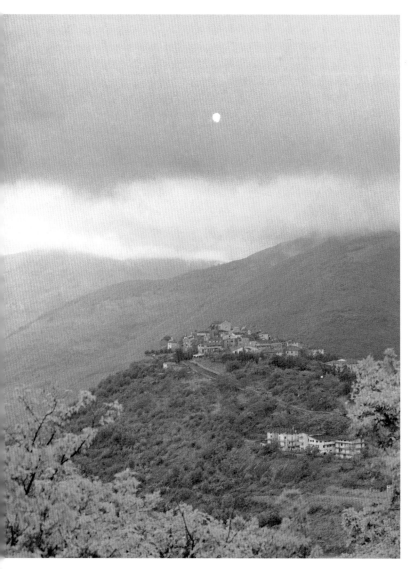

Campodimele was settled on an isolated mountain top in the eleventh century.

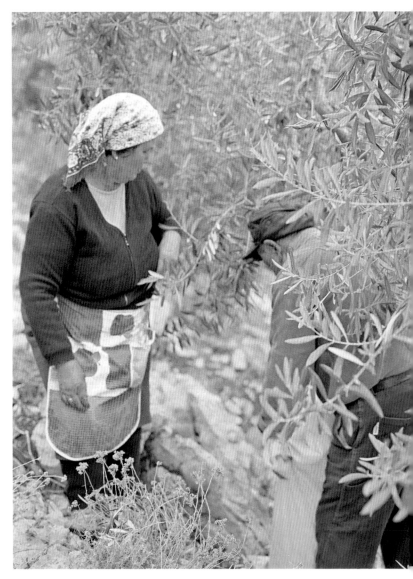

Maria and her family harvest their olive groves in the mountains, ensuring their annual supply of oil.

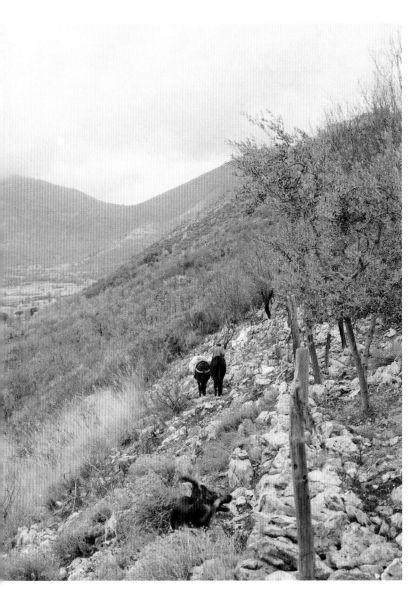

Four-legged transport is the only kind that can negotiate the terrain of Michele and Maria's olive terraces.

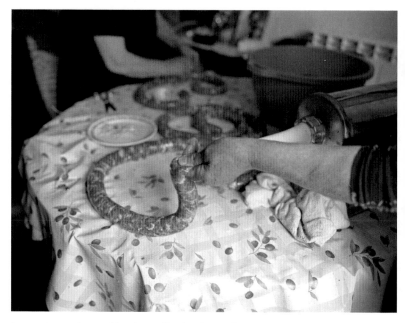

Leana maintains the age-old tradition of hand-making pork sausages (see page 30).

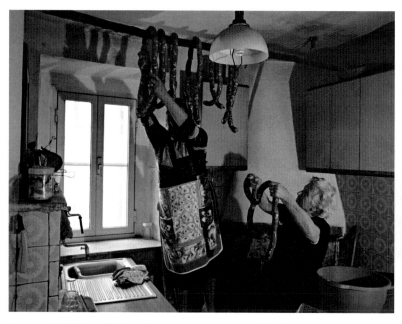

Assunta and Adelia hang freshly made sausages up to dry in Leana's kitchen.

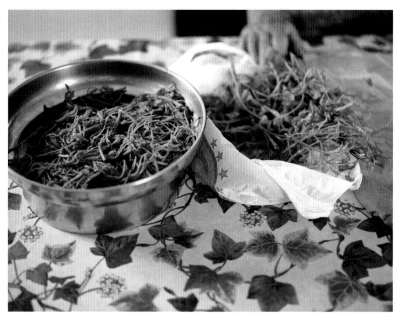

'Old man's beard', the wild clematis that villagers gather to make the *tagne* frittata.

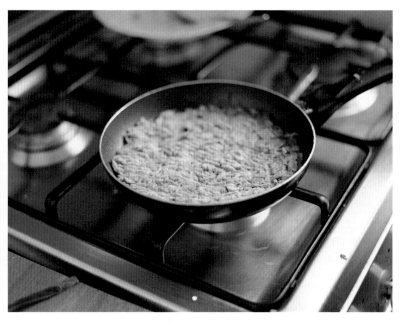

Tagne, the egg-free frittata that is a classic dish of Campodimele's *cucina povera* (see page 43).

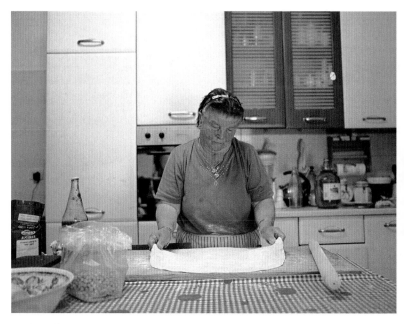

Natalina rolls hand-made pasta into leaves of lasagne (see page 51).

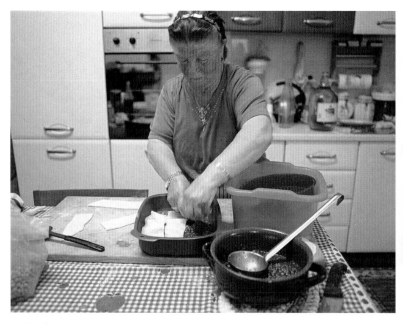

Natalina layers the pasta leaves, meat *ragù* and *fiordilatte* mozzarella to create her lasagne.

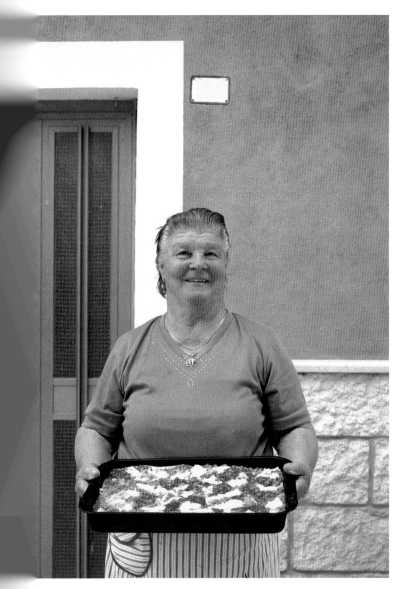

na holds her freshly baked lasagne outside her home.

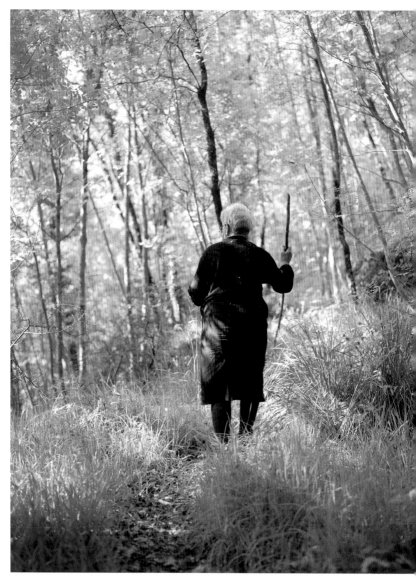

Adalgesia seeking wild asparagus in the woods.

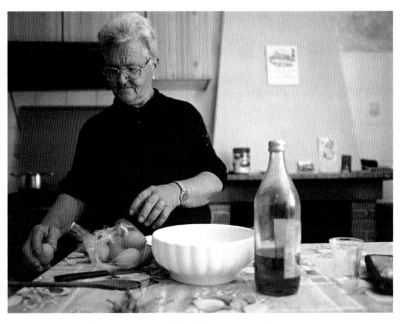

Adalgesia creating wild asparagus frittata in her kitchen (see page 43).

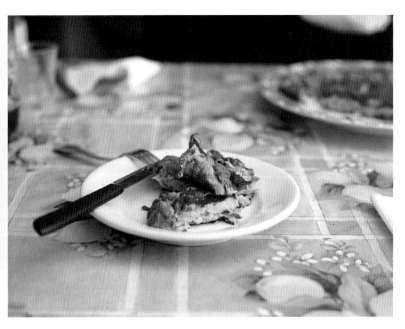

Wild asparagus frittata is a signature springtime dish of Campodimele.

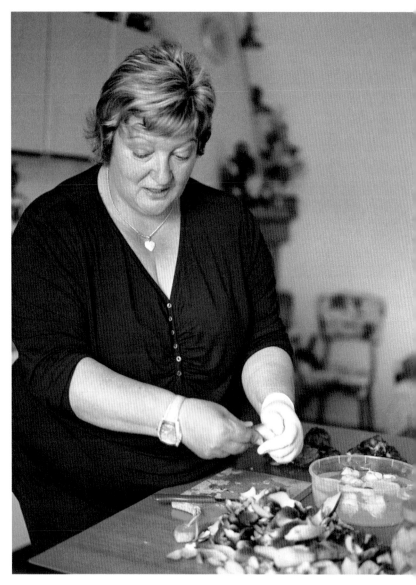

'Pina preparing *carciofini*, baby globe artichokes (see page 102).

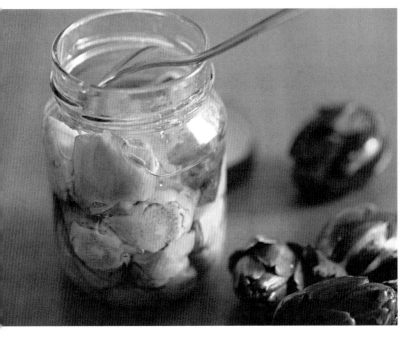

carciofini sott'olio – baby artichokes preserved under oil provide year-round antipasti (see page 106).

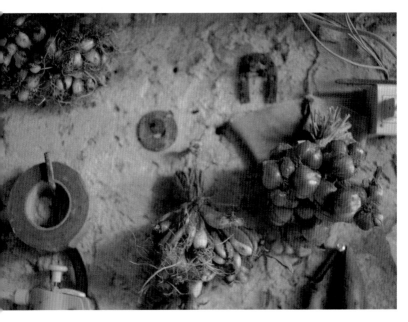

Seasonal gluts of food are conserved and stored in the *cantina*, the Italian larder.

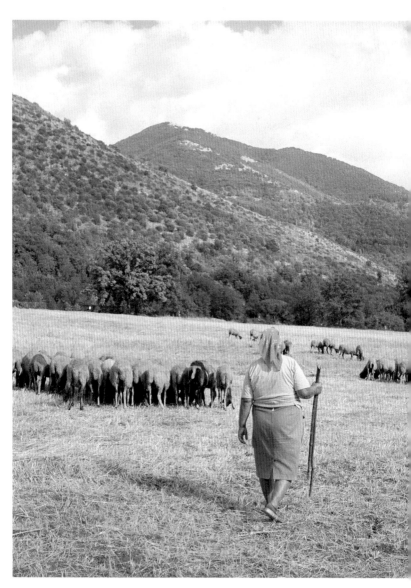

Maria Civita shepherding her sheep, as she has done all her life.

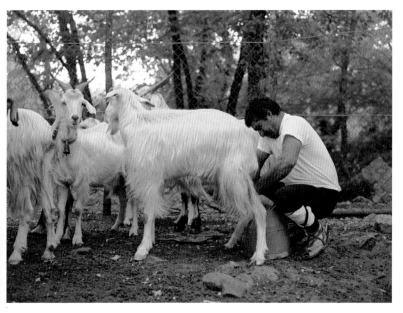

Adamo treads the mountainside with the help of *ciocce* – traditional shepherds' shoes made from fabric and car tyres.

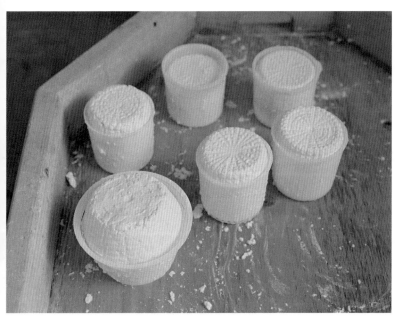

Milk from Adamo's goats has been handcrafted into cheese by his wife, Evelina.

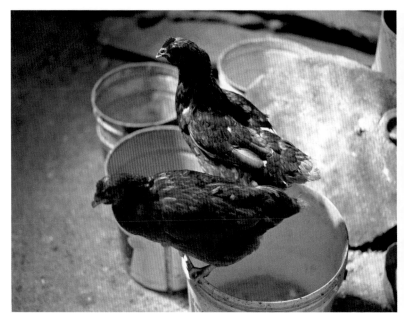

Le galline – the hens, which many of the older ladies keep to provide fresh, organic eggs for the table.

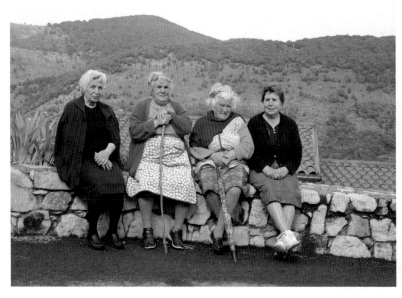

Pausing to chat after putting the hens to bed. Left to right: Adelia, Leana, Maria and Irma.

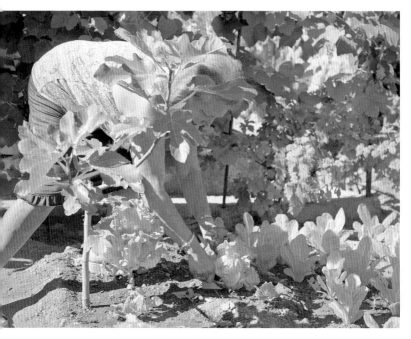

squalina picking fresh salad leaves in her *orto* for lunch.

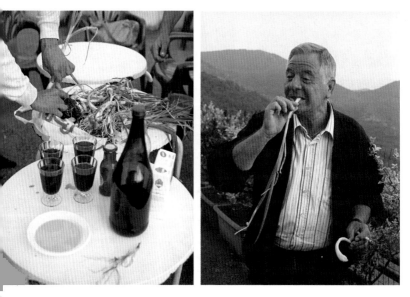

he first shallots are celebrated with *pinzimonio di scalogni* on the piazza – which Bruno is delighted to try.

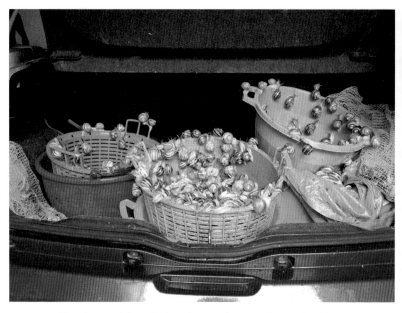

Ciamotte – wild snails – to celebrate the *festa* of San Onofrio, one of Campodimele's patron saints (see page 151).

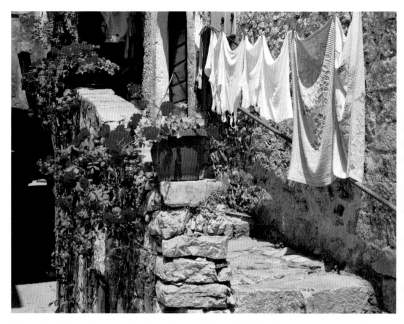

The medieval heart of Campodimele is a classic Italian rural idyll – eleventh-century stone houses and tumbling geraniums.

Stracciatella all'Assunta – Assunta's stracciatella

This soup does not look particularly appetizing, but it is worth getting past the visuals to enjoy its unusual texture and rich taste. This is sometimes served as a *primo* instead of *pasta in brodo* then followed by the chicken pieces as a main course.

1 litre (2 pints) chicken brodo, made according to the recipe
*   on page 59*
Four fresh organic eggs
200g (7oz) Parmigiano-Reggiano or Pecorino Romano,
*   freshly grated*
200g (7oz) freshly grated breadcrumbs
Fine sea salt

Put the *brodo* in a large pan and bring to a gentle simmer.

Meanwhile use a fork to thoroughly mix the eggs, cheese, breadcrumbs and a pinch of salt in a bowl.

Remove the *brodo* from the heat and gently pour in the egg mixture. Allow it to set for around one minute then stir to break up the eggs, and eat immediately.

Serves four.

Shallots on the Piazza

Italy is the land of the *sagre*, those annual festivals that celebrate the harvest of a particular food – be it tomatoes or almonds or oranges. But Italians do not need an official call to celebrate. A new crop is a chance to invite your neighbours for lunch and enjoy the first broad beans of the year; a sunny day is an excuse for a walk in the mountains and meat grilled over an open wood fire; the start of the hunting season is the moment to gather friends for dinner to share your first kill of the year.

When you produce as much of your own food as the Campomelani do, every week brings an opportunity for an unofficial *festa* like the one Attilio is organizing at the Moonlight Café tonight. This time it is the first *scalogni* out of the ground, the little shallots that are a signature note of Campomelano *cucina*. The excitement at table is palpable; everyone is talking about them. *Frittata agli scalogni* is a classic spring dish in these parts, I'm told – pan-fried eggs laced with sliced *scalogni* swimming in their own sugary juices. The bulbs can be dried and kept through the winter months, when they are added to soups rich with beans and pasta, a change from their cousin the onion. '*Un altro gusto!*' Attilio assures me, 'another taste. Like nothing you've ever eaten before.'

The mountains are already black against the apricot sky when we gather on the piazza, night creeping up on the *tramonto*, the 'between the mountains', which is how Italians describe the sunset. On the terrace of the café, Attilio has placed a white enamel table, bottles of red wine, glasses. Alongside them lie the much-anticipated *scalogni*, which he has procured with some trouble, because these early ones are so sought after. They don't look anything special – a bunch of muddy bulbs with long green tails, some of which have turned golden under the drying sun. They stink like sliced onions.

The men of the village are gathering to taste this seasonal treat. Brothers Patrizio, Elio and Norberto take the *scalogni* and one by one strip the outer layers and snap the roots from the bottom of the bulbs. Naked, they look like large spring onions, their white flesh glistening with moisture. Norberto squashes a bulb flat against a plate to release the juices, dips it in a dish of dressing – olive oil mixed with salt and white-wine vinegar – and offers it to me.

The raw *scalogno* is like a punch of acridity assaulting my tongue, its aftershock hitting my nose, bringing tears to my eyes. It's more bitter than the French shallots I am accustomed to, more pungent than an English spring onion. Just an hour or two out of the ground, the bulbs are still saturated with juice, and it feels as if the flavour will linger in my mouth for days.

'These are aphrodisiac,' Norberto assures me, but precisely who would be happy to get close to anyone who had snacked on raw *scalogno*, I can't imagine. Although it's clear they are an aid to sociability just now.

One by one, people wander over from the bar to squash a *scalogno*, dip it in *pinzimonio* dressing, crunch on the white bulb. They laugh at the pungency, swig a glass of red to mellow its strength, and now Bruno and Roberto are arguing over whether the *scalogni* have arrived a little early this year or at their usual time, the weather being so unusually warm and all. As the apricot sky fades to a soft purple, the truth about Italian food *sagre* is clearer than ever. Yes, they are about food; yes, they are about giving thanks for the new harvest; but just as much – perhaps even more – these *sagre* are about the fact that Italians love *stare in compagnia*, to enjoy company and commune with their fellow man.

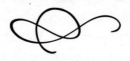

Pinzimonio di scalogni – Pinzimonio with shallots

Pinzimonio is the term used to describe any dish which uses seasoned olive oil as a dip for raw vegetables, and is a delicious antipasto. This also works well with sweet spring onions still on the stalk.

Bunch of fresh scalogni on the stalk
Good splash of extra-virgin olive oil
Splash of white-wine vinegar
Fine sea salt

Slice the bottoms from the *scalogni* bulbs and strip off the outer layer of skin, leaving a clean bulb.

Place the oil in a small bowl, add a splash of white-wine vinegar and a pinch of salt to taste then mix with a teaspoon.

Crush the raw *scalogni* bulbs against a flat surface, dip in the oil mixture and eat.

Frittata agli scalogni – Shallot omelette

The key to the success of this frittata is to fry the *scalogni
piano, piano*, 'gently, gently', over a very low heat, without
allowing them to colour, in order to release their sugary
juices. This recipe also works well with very finely sliced
golden onions. To make this frittata requires a 25 centimetre
(10 inch) pan with a non-stick surface.

*Ten scalogni bulbs, fresh or dried, or two large golden onions
Good splash of extra-virgin olive oil
Fine sea salt
Ten fresh organic eggs*

Peel the *scalogni* bulbs and slice them thinly widthways to
create small rounds.

Heat the olive oil in the frying pan then add the sliced
scalogni, along with two or three good pinches of salt.

Bring the contents of the pan to a high heat quickly then
turn the heat as low as possible and cook the *scalogni* gently
for around twenty minutes, stirring frequently and ensuring they do not brown.

While the *scalogni* are cooking, beat the eggs in a bowl.

When the *scalogni* are translucent and swimming in their
own juices, add the eggs and stir well to ensure the *scalogni*
are evenly distributed throughout the omelette mix.

Over a low heat, gently push the edges of the frittata
away from the sides and towards the middle of the pan,
continually tilting it to allow the liquid egg to run to the
edges and cook.

When most of the egg has solidified, lift the edge of the frittata to check that the underside is golden – once it is, cover the pan with a large plate and, holding the plate with the palm of one hand and the pan handle with the other, flip the pan upside down so the frittata drops onto the plate. Slide the frittata, uncooked side down, into the pan, and allow to cook for a few minutes more, until the underside is golden.

Slide onto a plate immediately. This is good served hot, but even better a few hours later, once the flavours of the *scalogni* have had time to mature.

Serves four to six.

Stracciatella agli scologni – Shallot soup streaked with eggs

Good splash of extra-virgin olive oil
Sixteen scalogni, sliced horizontally into rounds
Handful of fresh flat-leaf parsley, finely chopped
Two cloves of garlic, finely chopped
Fine sea salt
200ml (7fl oz) conserved tomato sauce (see page 263) or four
  fresh plum tomatoes, deseeded and chopped
1 litre (2 pints) chicken brodo, made according to the recipe
  on page 59 or vegetable stock
Four thick slices of stale, rough-textured bread, hand-cut
Four fresh organic eggs
200g (7oz) freshly grated Parmigiano-Reggiano or Pecorino
  Romano (optional)

Heat the oil in a large, deep pan. Cook the *scalogni* on a low heat for ten minutes, until translucent but not coloured.

Add the chopped parsley and garlic along with a pinch of salt, and cook for a minute further.

Add the sauce or tomatoes and simmer for a few minutes then add the stock and bring to a simmer. Set aside.

Place a slice of bread in the bottom of each of four serving bowls and splash with a little olive oil.

Beat the eggs in a bowl (along with the cheese, if using). Slowly pour the beaten egg mix into the soup. Allow to set for a minute then use a fork to gently break up the egg mix, into 'strings'.

Ladle the soup into each bowl over the bread and serve sprinkled with extra chopped parsley, if desired.

Serves four.

JUNE

Snails for San Onofrio

From up here you can't see the village, just the mountains rolling like rumpled velvet into the smooth expanse of the cerulean sky. And on a summer's day like this one, with only birdsong stirring the air, it's easy to understand why the Benedictines came here.

I'm standing at the gates of San Onofrio, the monastery situated high above Campodimele. In all the times I've come here, I've encountered only a handful of souls: a passing shepherd tending his sheep; the female cowherd droving her beautiful white cows; an occasional car carrying one of the few people who farm up here, or tourists exploring *Il Paese della Longevità*.

When the Benedictine monks created their community here almost a thousand years ago, it must have felt more isolated still – the perfect place to evoke the solitude of San Onofrio, the fifth-century saint who spent forty years in quiet contemplation in the Egyptian wilderness. The beauty of the landscape, the wisdom that comes with embracing Nature as your constant companion, were surely enough to give the friars the spiritual sustenance they sought. But how, I wonder, as I study the pale-stoned monastery and its gardens through the sun-warmed bars of the iron gates, how did they sustain their more earthly needs?

Campodimele is a good two-hour walk away on a mountain path, so when the Benedictines first settled here, they would have needed to be self-sufficient in a way which wouldn't be necessary today. No doubt they farmed an *orto* and kept hens and goats. And maybe they braved the brigand-infested hills to gather wild asparagus and trap hare and boar. In summer, I wonder, did they gather *ciammotte*, wild snails from the beech woods, and serve them dressed in *salsa verde* on 12 June, the feast of San Onofrio, a tradition the villagers will celebrate tomorrow?

I catch the scent of mint and garlic even before Adalgesia opens her farmhouse door. A whiff of wood-smoke too. She's been up since 4.00 a.m., she tells me, as she kisses me once on each cheek and draws me into the warmth of her kitchen.

It's now after 6.00 a.m. and the purple June night is ceding to the summer dawn, but the gossamer mist of the rising dew carries a damp chill, and it feels wonderful to sit by Adalgesia's stove, absorbing the heat from its gas flames and the aroma from the Moka pot in which the espresso is brewing.

Early starts are a way of life for Adalgesia. In summers past, the men would walk out to their fields while it was still dark and work from first light to midday, when the sun drove them home to lunch and a siesta. On short winter days, before electricity, every hour of daylight was needed. Rising with the sun, retiring as night falls: a rhythm in sync with Nature which may, studies suggest, aid longevity due to its impact on melatonin levels in the body.

'*Le ciammotte,*' Adalgesia says, as she lifts the lid from a pan simmering on the cooker to reveal a pile of brindled brown spirals. The shells are flecked with the green of spring garlic tails and the fresh wild mint whose perfume scents the fields these damp summer mornings.

Ciammotte are, it seems, the traditional San Onofrio dish because there is an abundance of them in the fields just now. Adalgesia hasn't gathered these herself, but – like most people today – buys them from an enterprising soul who lives outside the village and harvests them high in the surrounding hills, managing to sell them only because people trust that these are wild snails, as opposed to farmed ones. They are, however, the only ingredient of the San Onofrio lunch which Adalgesia has bought – everything else she has grown or gathered herself.

After the snails will come the *caprettone*, the five-month-old goat Adalgesia killed and jointed at 5.30 this morning, before the flies were out and about. It's marinating in olive oil, rosemary, parsley and garlic, and will cook *alla brace* outside. Adalgesia will serve the goat with a *contorno* of leafy *broccoletti*, which she froze when it was abundant in her winter *orto*, and a frittata laced with wild asparagus, also gathered and frozen in the spring. Melding the old ways of preserving with the new, I think to myself.

Now she is chopping three plum tomatoes and adding them to the snails with another vigorous *mescolata*, a good mix with a wooden spoon. A little longer and the snails will be ready. By the time Adalgesia's family arrive for lunch, they will have cooled, their flesh relaxed and ready to eat. Many people eat snails cold, not least because it is more convenient to cook them in advance. But they are good hot, I discover, as I tease one from its shell with the tine of a fork, and taste the saltiness of the garlic fighting with the sweet high notes of the mint. I wonder if it was the Benedictines who started this tradition of eating snails for the feast of San Onofrio. If so, did they eat them hot or cold? And dressed in mountain herbs?

Weeks pass. It's the end of June, and I'm at San Onofrio again, but not alone. Usually the monastery church is only open to the public by appointment, but traditionally, on 30 June, a special Mass is held in honour of this patron saint, followed by three more Masses mid-month in July, August and September. The church's beauty lies in its simplicity – plain lines, white walls, a simple altar and a statue of the saint, his long white beard symbolizing his four decades in the desert.

It took us twenty-five minutes to drive up the steep and stony mountain path – Pasqualina, Assunta, Marietta and me, my driving as slow as a *ciammotta*, we laugh. When they were children they used to make the pilgrimage by foot. '*Ci voleva tanto tempo!*' It took so much time.

Outside the monastery villagers are gathered, reciting the rosary – the same prayers the Benedictines would have offered daily here.

As we file into the church, I spot Adalgesia and thank her again for my wonderful San Onofrio's lunch. And it strikes me that, a thousand years after the Benedictines came to these parts, Adalgesia's kitchen is almost as self-sufficient as the monastery's must have been then – but because she prefers to live that way, not because it has to be.

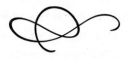

Ciammotte alla salsa verde —Wild snails in green sauce

First you need to catch your snails! Or buy them, live, from a reputable supplier. If you are lucky, your snail-catcher will purge them for you – that is, clear out the snails' digestive systems so they are safe to eat. If you need to purge them yourself, keep them in a well-ventilated cage for several days and feed them on plain flour, ensuring they have a fresh and plentiful water supply. After five days – maybe more – the snails should pass only the white flour, at which point you can be sure they are purged and ready to eat.

1 kg (2lb 3oz) purged snails, live
Few splashes of extra-virgin olive oil
Handful of fresh flat-leaf parsley, finely chopped
Two heads of fresh garlic or four large cloves of garlic,
*   finely chopped*
Two green tails of fresh garlic, finely chopped
Handful of celery leaves, finely chopped
Handful of fresh mint, finely chopped
Several pinches of fine sea salt
Two plum tomatoes, finely chopped

Rinse the purged snails well in lots of cold water and scrub their shells clean.

Gently heat the olive oil in a large, deep pan big enough to accommodate all the snails easily.

Add the chopped parsley, garlic, garlic tails and celery leaves, and fry very gently for a minute or two, making sure that the garlic does not colour or burn. Add the chopped mint to the other ingredients already in the pan.

Now add the snails, and fill the pan with enough cold water to just cover them.

Add three or four good pinches of salt, and stir gently so that the *odori* are well distributed.

Gently bring the water to the boil – this should make the snails emerge from their shells, which will make them easy to access later.

Cover the pan, and simmer gently for around two hours, stirring frequently. During this time, the water should evaporate, leaving the snails to steam in their oily sauce.

After about two hours, add the chopped tomatoes and mix well, cover the pan again, and allow to cook gently for a further fifteen minutes.

Now remove one of the snails from the pan, and, spearing the fleshy part with a toothpick, separate it from its shell and taste it – the snail should be softly edible, not rubbery.

Mix well and serve hot or cold, slicked with some of the sauce.

Serves six to eight.

Caprettone alla brace – Baby goat cooked over charcoal

If you are lucky enough to have a wood-burning open fire, reduce the wood to charcoal before cooking the goat; otherwise you can use a domestic barbecue.

Good splash of extra-virgin olive oil
Handful of fresh flat-leaf parsley sprigs
Couple of rosemary sprigs, halved, but with the leaves still attached
Four cloves of garlic, peeled and squashed against the side of a knife
2kg (4lb 6oz) goat pieces, on the bone

Mix the oil, herbs, garlic and goat meat in a bowl, and place somewhere cool to marinate for a few hours – or in the fridge overnight.

If the meat has been in the fridge overnight, remove at least half an hour before cooking, so it can return to room temperature.

When the charcoal is ready, place the meat in a barbecue grill pan and position it in the hearth, close to, but not touching, the embers for about ten to fifteen minutes on each side. Alternatively place on a barbecue until cooked through.

Serves six to eight.

Spaghetti con sugo di pomodoro e pollo — Spaghetti in tomato and chicken sugo

Another two-in-one recipe. The tomato sauce emerges flavoured with the chicken pieces and is used to dress the pasta for the *primo*; the chicken pieces are set aside and eaten with the *secondo* or immediately after the pasta.

Good splash of extra-virgin olive oil
One medium-sized golden onion, finely chopped
One stick of celery and leaves, finely chopped
Few sprigs of fresh flat-leaf parsley, finely chopped
Four chicken wings or thighs
Fine sea salt
Medium-sized glass of good dry white wine
1 litre (2 pints) conserved tomato sauce (see page 263)
400g (14oz) dried spaghetti

Heat the oil in a wide, deep pan then gently fry the onion and celery for around ten minutes, ensuring the onion does not brown.

Add the chopped parsley, and cook for a minute or two.

Add the chicken pieces, and fry gently for a minute or so on each side.

Add two or three good pinches of salt and the white wine, bring to the boil then reduce the heat and allow to simmer for a few minutes until the wine is reduced.

Add the tomato sauce, bring the pan to the boil then lower the heat and simmer gently, partially covered, for around forty minutes.

When the chicken is thoroughly cooked, remove the pan from the heat and place the chicken on a plate, wrapped in aluminium foil.

Bring a large pan of salted water to the boil and cook the spaghetti according to the instructions on the packet – usually eight to ten minutes. When it is cooked, drain and throw it into the pan of tomato sauce. Stir gently to coat every strand and serve immediately.

Serves four.

Every Part of the Plant

Zucchine are the most extravagant of plants: rampant jungles of lush green leaves, flourishing trumpets of golden flowers, an endless abundance of glossy fruits.

Examining Amalia's *zucchine* in the *orto* behind her house, I can see their beauty, but the fruit has never captured my heart. Too often I find *zucchine* to be a bland vehicle for the herbs in which they are dressed, fruits lacking a taste of their own; spongy, watery flesh covered by skin with a bitter tang.

But in Campodimele they are one of the first crops of the summer *orto*, and, watching them run wild among the orderly rows of lettuce and beans, I couldn't help wondering if their *gioia di vivere*, their joy for life, might improve their taste.

'*Ogni parte della pianta*,' says Amalia, washing the freshly plucked courgettes in her kitchen sink, 'every part of the plant. That's the beauty of the *zucchina*. You can use the flesh, the small leaves, even the stalk. And, of course, you can eat the flowers.'

It's the flowers which have seduced me into giving *zucchine* a second chance: outsized yellow stars spangling under the sun. *Zucchina* flowers are sold still attached to the slender green batons of fruit here, or in bundles on their own. Their trumpet shape is perfect for stuffing, perhaps with ricotta, a little dried chilli, a sun-dried tomato or two. Fold the petals over the filling and serve raw, or dip in batter and fry in olive oil. The fried flowers have a green sweetness and are crispy in the mouth, perfect packaging for melting cheese, delicious enough to justify growing the plants without bothering with the green fruits. But Amalia insists that her *zucchina* fruits are good too – along with the leaves and the stalks, which certainly sound worth a try.

The simplest way to enjoy every part of this plant is in a *minestra*. It seems Amalia's entire summer *orto* is already cooking in this pan of soup: onions, garlic, tomatoes, flat green *coralli* beans in their pods, a few fresh borlotti beans, diced potatoes. She chops the *zucchine*, their thin stalks and their curly little leaves, and adds them to the mix. Then she picks up the flowers, plucks out their pollen-bearing pistils and throws the petals into the bubbling soup. They look so delicate I fear they'll dissolve, but they don't. And here's a piece of raw *zucchina* left over on the side. I bite into it and it's like eating a fruit I've never tried before: the flesh has a tight-textured crunch, a creamy freshness, with no chemical tang in the skin. But what about when they are cooked?

We eat the minestrone cold the next day, a cooling first course for a summer lunch. It's perfect: the flavours of each component have melded in the broth, but each vegetable, pulse and fruit retains a taste of its own. The *zucchina* flowers are sweet in the mouth, the leaves have a dark depth, and I can sense the crunch of the sliced stalks in every spoonful. But what about the flesh? I fish a piece out with my spoon and give it a try. It's good. Still crunchy, creamy, fresh on the tongue. Every part of the plant indeed. Bursting with *gioia di vivere*.

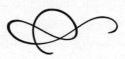

Minestra ai fiori di zucchine – Zucchina flower soup

If you are lucky enough to be able to find *zucchine* complete
with their flowers, leaves and stalks, use every part of the
plant to make this soup.

Good splash of extra-virgin olive oil
One large golden onion, finely sliced
Handful of fresh flat-leaf parsley, chopped
Two cloves of garlic, finely chopped
Two large potatoes, diced
Handful of fresh, podded borlotti beans
Handful of flat green coralli beans, or string beans, sliced
300ml (10fl oz) conserved tomato sauce (see page 263)
Fine sea salt
Four small zucchine plus their flowers, along with four more
    zucchina flowers – remove the pistils, the internal stalks,
    of the flowers, and discard them
Handful of zucchina stalks and leaves, if available
100g (3½oz) Parmigiano-Reggiano or Pecorino Romano,
    finely grated

Heat the olive oil in a large deep pan, and fry the onion
gently for about ten minutes, until it is translucent but not
coloured.

Add the parsley, garlic and diced potatoes and fry for a
minute or so, ensuring the garlic does not burn.

Add the borlotti beans, the sliced coralli or string beans,
the tomato conserve and a couple of good pinches of salt
to taste.

Next add enough cold water to the pan to cover the vegetables by a few centimetres, bring to the boil, lower the heat and simmer, partially covered, for about 20 minutes.

Chop the *zucchine* into cubes about 2cm (1in) square, and chop their stalks and leaves, if using.

Leave the flowers whole. Add all of the *zucchina* pieces, stir, and simmer for a further 25 minutes, or until the borlotti beans are tender.

Serve hot, scattered with the grated cheese, or serve cold, or reheated, the next day.

Serves four to six.

Zucchine alla parmigiana – Fried zucchine with Parmesan

It's important to use a large pan when frying *zucchine* to ensure they fry rather than steam in the large amount of water they contain. If you have a small pan, cook this in two batches. These are also delicious straight from the pan, without the Parmesan cheese, if you prefer.

Four zucchine
Good splash of extra-virgin olive oil
One clove of garlic, finely chopped
Handful of fresh flat-leaf parsley, finely chopped
Fine sea salt
100g (3½oz) Parmigiano-Reggiano cheese, freshly grated

Preheat the oven to 200°C/400°F/Gas Mark 6.

Slice the *zucchine* into flat discs, on the diagonal.

Heat the olive oil in a large frying pan and when it is very hot, sauté the garlic gently for about 20 seconds then fling in the *zucchine* and fry over a good heat for a minute or two until they just begin to turn gold on each side.

Stir in the parsley and salt to taste then tip the *zucchine* into an oven-proof baking dish and scatter over the grated cheese.

Place the dish in the preheated oven for 15 minutes, or until the cheese has melted and is golden on top.

Serves three as a main course, five as a side dish.

Fiori di zucchina ripieni – Stuffed zucchina flowers

Twelve zucchina flowers
600g (1lb 5oz) ricotta
Splash of extra-virgin olive oil
Four sun-dried tomatoes cut into fine strips
Handful of fresh flat-leaf parsley, finely chopped
Fine sea salt
Crushed dried red chilli (optional)

Trim the *zucchina* flowers and remove and discard the pistils – the stalks within the flower head.

In a bowl, mix the ricotta with a splash of olive oil, the sun-dried tomato strips, the parsley, two or three pinches of salt, and a couple of pinches of dried chilli, if using.

Peel back the petals of the *zucchina* flowers, making sure not to tear them, then lay the flower head on its side. Spread a spoonful of the cheese mixture onto one petal, add another, then carefully close the petals around the stuffing and place on a serving plate.

Serve as antipasti, with a glass of good white wine.

Makes twelve stuffed flowers.

Zucchine fritte in pastella alla birra –
Zucchine fried in beer batter

Vegetables fried in batter are often prepared in advance in Campodimele and served at room temperature rather than hot.

100g (3½oz) '00' Doppio Zero flour or plain flour
250ml (½ pint) Italian beer – Nastro Azzurro is very popular around here
One fresh organic egg
Fine sea salt
Four small zucchine
Good splash of extra-virgin olive oil

In a large bowl beat together the flour, beer, egg and a couple of good pinches of sea salt and leave to stand for around 30 minutes.

Meanwhile slice the *zucchine* thinly, on the diagonal, and sprinkle with a little salt.

When the batter has rested for 30 minutes, heat the olive oil in a pan and tip the *zucchine* into the batter, making sure each one is well coated.

When the oil is very hot, spoon the battered *zucchine* into it and fry until golden on the underside, then flip the *zucchine* over and fry on the other side until golden.

Place on a plate lined with kitchen paper to soak up any excess oil, and serve hot or at room temperature.

July

Out of the Woods

So much of the Campodimele *cucina* begins here: on the eastern slopes of the oak grove, amid the whisper of the western breeze, hundreds of metres above Campodimele's historic core.

It's 7.00 on a July morning and the sun spills like lava over the mountain summits, flickering like a flame up the skinny tree trunks and flashing fire amid the foliage. Down behind the village walls, the cool of the night still lingers, but up here, on the open hill, the fierce heat of summer is already felt.

To get here, you have to ditch the car seven kilometres up the mountain road that winds behind Campodimele and walk a few hundred metres along a stone-strewn track until you reach a clearing in the woods. Carry on uphill until the forest floor spews up its chalk rocks and you're in the heart of the *cerreto*, the oak grove. The way ahead isn't clear, but if you stop for a moment and catch the breath of the breeze, you can hear the jangle of the bells, guiding you on.

The bells are worn by the horses, and, as you scramble higher, you find them waiting for you, curious chestnut heads craning from behind trees, ears pricked towards your unfamiliar footsteps. Only once they've checked you out do they step into view, and that's when you see the logs strapped to their sides.

These are the horses that carry the wood that fires the ovens on which the Campomelani cook much of their food. Without the horses there would be no logs because wheeled vehicles can't negotiate this terrain. Without the logs there would be no *forno a legna* in which to bake pizza and bread. No *fuochi*, the open-hearth fires where pulses simmer to a smoky mustiness. And no *brace* of crumbled charcoal to grill meat. So in one sense, the *raccolta di legna*, the wood harvest, is where much of the cooking begins.

The *raccolta* is organized by the Comune di Campodimele, the local council, and starts in November, when the mountains are bathed in mist and rain. Over the eight months that follow, the team of forest workers cuts by chainsaw 10,000 *quintali* of oak logs – more than 950,000 kilos. They strap the wood in bundles to the flanks of the horses and send them down the mountains with a slap on the rump and a cry of '*Su, muoviti!*' – 'On you go!'

There are eight horses and this year a foal who trots after his mother as she works her way up and down the mountain. There's Toby, the leader, who might nuzzle his velvet lips against your hand as he passes by. Then Silvana, Bimba, Pupa, Rondinella, Giulia, Vespa, Bionda and her baby, Bello. They make their way down the mountain one by one, without any human guide, until they come to the clearing, and here the workers unstrap the logs. Then the horses form a line, waiting to be roped together and led back up the mountain to the spot where the next load of logs is already being felled. The wood they carry is sold to the villagers, who store them in their *cantine* and outhouses. Even on the hottest days of summer you can see the womenfolk carrying wood piled high on their heads through the streets to fuel the *forni* and fires with which meals will be cooked.

So in a sense this is the beginning, but today it is also an ending, because this first Saturday in July marks the last day of this season's *raccolta di legna*. It's a day to take stock of another successful year of wood collecting and to give thanks for another harvest safely home. It's a day to celebrate the horses without whom the fires and *forni* would go unlit. A day for the forest workers and men and boys of the village to gather for an al fresco *festa*.

If you leave the horses high on the mountain and scramble back down, you find that the clearing in the woods has been transformed. A green net suspended from the oak branches creates a shady roof over a trestle table around which are ranged white plastic chairs for forty people. Now the breeze brings you the smoky-sweet mix of wood roasting, charcoal burning and meat cooking, and if you follow the scent you find the *festa* has begun.

The open grill is heavy with meat – *salsiccia piccante*, fresh pork sausage laced with hot chilli pepper; *carne*, the word for 'meat' which is used to describe beef in these parts; *maiale*, pork fillet, which today has been marinated in rosemary and garlic before being flung over the flames. These are already being eaten by the forest workers, who have been on the hill since dawn. Later more meat will be grilled for the festive lunch. The highlight of the meal will be the goat stew being cooked further down the mountain, at the home of the shepherd who has killed the animal. It will be brought up by car when it's ready to eat. Its sauce will dress the pasta for the *primo*, the chunks of meat serving as *secondo*.

The diners are arriving now, in twos and threes: old men who've been working their fields, accompanied by their sons and their grandsons; the park rangers who manage the flora and fauna of the Aurunci Mountains; members of the local council. Friends, neighbours, colleagues, coming together to celebrate the fruits of the foresters' labour. The trestle table is laid with white picnic plates, cutlery and beakers; the guests are eating antipasti of olives and cheese, quaffing red wine with its edge of roughness – the best wine for drinking with wood-smoked meat. There is laughter, joking and, as always at Italian gather-ings over food, a tangible air of anticipation of the delights to come: reminiscences about how good the goat sauce was at last year's *festa*, predictions of how delicious it is sure to taste today.

Dressed in a white chef's hat, Luigi Papa is tending the grill while keeping an eye on a metallic vat of salted water bubbling over an open fire. The goat sauce is on its way, and the water must be ready for the 6 kilos of pasta that will cook in the 15 litres of water. He shows me the spoon he will use to stir the pasta – it has a hook for hanging carved onto its handle in the traditional Campodimele style. It's aged beyond memory, having belonged to Luigi's mother, and huge – over 70 centimetres long: a spoon from a fairy tale.

The sauce is good – everyone agrees. The tomato base is thick with parsley and onion, the gamey flavour of goat clinging to every strand of pasta. The next course is even better – chunks of goat meat, much of it still on the bone, dark with the flavour of mountain grass, sweet at the fatty edges.

Refreshing green salad, bowls of fresh fruit, sweet *crostate*, the huge flat pastry tarts filled with *amarene*, apricot, chocolate spread – the feast follows the familiar pattern of long Italian lunches. The outdoor setting lends itself perfectly to the conviviality of celebration. The sun soars high then sinks low, and soon will be setting not just on this *festa* but on this season's wood harvest. Through the trees come the bells of the horses who will be led into the clearing to receive applause from the men who've celebrated their work under the summer sun today. Later they will be set free to wander the mountains through the summer months; you'll come across them resting in the shade of the leafy canopies, crossing your path on the track up to San Onofrio. Until autumn comes again, and the hearth fires must be fuelled every day, and the horses return to the harvest.

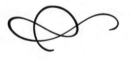

Primo di pappardelle al sugo di capra e secondo di capra —
Pasta ribbons dressed in goat-meat sauce
followed by goat stew

In this two-in-one dish, the *odori* are the foreground taste in the pasta dish, with the meat offering background notes, while in the *secondo*, the meat is the star, with the herbs in which it was cooked providing enhancement. Goat stew was traditionally eaten at wedding feasts in Campodimele.

1.5kg (3lb 5oz) goat pieces — shank on the bone and neck cuts are good for this dish
Three good splashes of extra-virgin olive oil
Two medium-sized golden onions, finely chopped
Six sprigs of flat-leaf parsley
Large splash of good white wine
Fine sea salt
One quantity of fresh egg pappardelle ribbons, made according to the recipe on page 55, or 400g (14oz) dried pappardelle
1 litre (2 pints) conserved tomato sauce (see page 263)

The taste of goat meat can be a little overpowering sometimes, so to avoid this, first help the meat to *cacciare l'acqua* – literally 'to chase its water', so emitting much of its fluid content and strong flavour. To do this, place the meat in a deep, broad-based pan along with a glass or two of water.

Bring to the boil then simmer gently for around twenty to thirty minutes.

Remove the meat, discard the cooking water, and rinse and dry the pan.

Now heat the oil in the pan, and, when it is hot, fry the onion and parsley sprigs for a few minutes over a high heat – but do not allow them to brown.

Replace the meat in the pan, and fry quickly over a high heat for a few minutes on each side, until it is browned.

Add the wine, simmering for a few minutes until reduced.

Add enough water to barely cover the meat, along with three or four good pinches of salt. Raise the heat until the water begins to simmer then lower the heat, cover with a lid, and allow to cook very gently for around ninety minutes, stirring and turning the pieces of meat occasionally.

If using freshly made *pappardelle*, begin to make them now, according to the instructions on page 57; this will allow time for resting and cutting before the goat stew is ready. Once you have cut the ribbons, dust them with flour, and cover with a clean tea towel.

When the goat meat feels fork-tender, add the tomato sauce and cook gently for a further forty or so minutes. If the sauce begins to look dry, add a little cold water to thin it out. Remove the meat from the pan to a warmed serving dish, and keep it warm.

Now use the sauce to coat the pasta. Bring a large pan of salted water to the boil, and cook the fresh egg *pappardelle* ribbons for two or three minutes until they are al dente – or cook the dried *pappardelle* according to the instructions on the packet. Drain the pasta, and tip it into the pan of sauce, stirring gently so every strand is coated. Serve in warm bowls.

Serve the goat meat as the second course, along with lots of crusty bread and some wilted green vegetables such as *broccoletti* or *cicoria* greens.

Serves four to six.

Maiale alla griglia con rosmarino e aglio –
Grilled pork fillet marinated in rosemary and garlic

Alla griglia means 'barbecued', but this dish is also delicious cooked under a conventional grill.

Two splashes of extra-virgin olive oil
Four cloves of garlic, finely sliced
Two sprigs of rosemary, crushed
Four pork fillets

Place the oil, garlic and rosemary in a shallow dish along with the pork, ensuring the pork is bathed all over with the oil.

Cover and leave in the fridge for at least two hours, turning occasionally.

Half an hour before cooking, remove the meat from the fridge and allow it to return to room temperature.

Cook on the barbecue for three or four minutes on each side, or until cooked through.

Serves four.

Potatoes Like Parsley

'*Prezzemolo!*' everyone exclaims, 'Parsley!' – although it's not parsley we are talking about. You put them in the ground, then you forget about them, then whatever you dig up – '*Prezzemolo!*' You sit down for lunch and – '*Prezzemolo!*'

I need to turn to the dictionary for help on this one. '*Essere come il prezzemolo*', says my heavyweight volume of the Garzanti Hazon wordbook, is an idiom that translates literally as 'to be like parsley' – by which the Italians mean something or someone inclined to turn up everywhere. That's why they describe potatoes as *prezzemolo*.

I hadn't expected to find potatoes in such abundance in the Campodimele *cucina*, not least because when I first came here and fell into discussions about the differences between British and Italian cuisine, people always asked if it was true that my fellow *inglesi* eat a lot of potatoes. The traditional British diet includes almost as many potatoes as the Italian diet contains pasta, I'd reply, never gaining any inkling that on tables here, *patate* also turn up all the time and everywhere. But I think it's fair to say that the Campomelani are more imaginative in their day-to-day use of potatoes than many of my fellow Brits.

Here potatoes might be boiled and mashed and mixed with flour to make gnocchi, the little dumplings often served as a *primo* in place of pasta, but they might also be diced and fried gently with *odori* of onion, garlic, celery leaf and tomato to form a thick vegetable stock in which pasta is boiled to create the simplest, most satisfying soup. Potatoes are often added whole to a mixed-vegetable minestrone and, once cooked, mashed with a fork to thicken the mix.

But such is their exquisite sweetness here that I believe they are at their best when they are the key taste of a dish: sliced and fried gently in the incomparably fruity local extra-virgin olive oil; chopped and mixed with whole garlic cloves, rosemary sprigs, salt and olive oil, and baked in the oven until their flesh turns to a creamy meltedness.

Potatoes thrive here and they could never be described as bland. They grow in pure earth which has never known chemical treatment; they are encouraged with natural animal fertilizers. There is nothing artificial to mask the flavour of these tubers.

My friend Pasquale grows potatoes in the garden of his house in the *centro storico*: a bit of soil, a bit of sun, a bit of rain, and they flourish and spread underground with an abundance which even their rich forest of green leaves barely betrays. His father and grandfather grew potatoes here before him. Now he stoops and gives a sharp tug to one of the plants. The potatoes fly out like a cache of long-lost treasures: a golden cascade mottled with soil. If we dig beneath the leafy forests of the *zucchina* leaves, we'll probably find others. And buried beneath the onions too.

Potatoes are sown in October for a July harvest, but like so many things which earn a space in the *orto*, they are a store-cupboard food too. Kept in Pasquale's *cantina* or *magazzino*, these potatoes will still be good to eat eight or nine months from now, in any number of dishes: as rampant at the table as *prezzemolo*.

Pasquale loves to eat them in their simplest state: wrapped in silver foil then baked gently beneath the *cenere*, the cinders of the wood fire he sets in his fireplace, their skins smoked and crisped. He also enjoys them as *panzerotti*, the Campomelano croquettes which his wife, Amalia, makes. '*Lei sa fare tutto!*' he enthuses. 'She knows how to do everything!' He talks with the Italian male's unabashed pride in his womenfolk's cooking skills. '*Lei ha le mani sante!*' – 'She has blessed hands!'

I agree with him – Amalia's cooking is fit for angels. To make her meltingly delicious *panzerotti* she boils potatoes and squeezes them through a potato ricer, then mixes them with Parmesan, salt and eggs before forming them into small sausages, which she dips in egg and breadcrumbs and fries in her home-produced olive oil. But her *panzerotto* mix is not complete unless she steps out into her kitchen *orto* and snaps off a stalk or two of the green herb that marries perfectly with her potatoes and turns up everywhere in this *cucina – prezzemolo*.

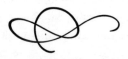

Patate con fagiolini – Potato and green-bean salad

800g (2lb) potatoes suitable for boiling
400g (14oz) long green beans (French beans)
Good splash of extra-virgin olive oil
Juice of half a lemon
Two cloves of garlic, finely sliced
Fine sea salt
Handful of fresh flat-leaf parsley, finely chopped

Scrub the potatoes clean then, leaving their skins on, place them in a large pan of well-salted cold water and bring to the boil. Boil for around twenty minutes, or until the centres are tender to the point of a sharp knife.

While the potatoes are boiling, top and tail the green beans then place them into a large pan of boiling salted water for twenty to thirty minutes, until they are soft to the bite. Drain in a colander and refresh with cold water.

To make the dressing, mix together the olive oil, lemon juice, sliced garlic and sea salt to taste.

Drain the potatoes, and, when they are cool enough to handle, peel away the skins if preferred and cut the flesh into small chunks.

Place the potatoes in a bowl along with the green beans, pour over the dressing then sprinkle over the chopped parsley. Stir well, coating all the potatoes in the dressing to prevent them discolouring. This tastes better if allowed to rest for at least half an hour, so the potatoes can absorb the flavours.

Serves four to six.

Panzerotti – Potato and cheese croquettes

Campomelano cooks boil potatoes in their skins, to help prevent them becoming waterlogged. When doing this it is important to choose potatoes of the same size, to ensure they all cook at the same rate. Potatoes boiled in their skins also require more salt after they have been peeled than those boiled in salted water without their skins.

1kg (2lb 3oz) potatoes suitable for boiling
Fine sea salt
Four large, fresh organic eggs
150g (5oz) Parmigiano-Reggiano or Pecorino Romano, freshly grated
Handful of fresh flat-leaf parsley, finely chopped
About 250g (9oz) fresh breadcrumbs
Handful of plain flour
Three or four splashes of extra-virgin olive oil

Scrub the potatoes, and, leaving them in their skins, place them in a large pan of well-salted cold water and bring to the boil.

Boil the potatoes for around twenty minutes, or until the centres are tender when tested with the point of a sharp knife.

Drain the potatoes and, when cool enough to handle, remove and discard their skins. Press the peeled potatoes through a potato ricer into a large bowl – or place straight in the bowl and mash finely with a potato masher.

Now, beat two of the eggs together in a bowl.

Add the beaten eggs to the potatoes, add three or four good pinches of salt, and mix using a fork. Then add the grated cheese and the parsley, and mix well.

Now beat the remaining two eggs in a bowl, and pour the breadcrumbs into a separate shallow dish. Scatter the flour onto a flat work surface.

To structure the *panzerotti*, take small lumps of the potato mixture – about the size of a golf ball – and, on the floured work surface, roll them into small sausage shapes, flattening the ends.

When all the potato mixture has been shaped into sausages, one by one roll them in the egg, then dip them in the breadcrumbs and set aside.

Heat the olive oil in a large frying pan, and, when it is hot, place about half of the *panzerotti* into the pan and fry gently on a low heat, turning frequently, for around seven minutes, or until the breadcrumbs are crispy and golden. Use tongs to stand the croquettes on each of their flat ends for a moment or two to ensure they are cooked and golden all over.

Remove to a plate covered with kitchen paper to absorb any excess oil.

Clean the pan to remove overcooked breadcrumbs, add another splash of olive oil, and cook the remaining *panzerotti* in the same way. These are delicious hot, but also very good served at room temperature.

Makes around sixteen croquettes.

Pasta con le patate – Pasta and potato soup

The notion of putting pasta and potatoes together may seem strange at first, but this hearty soup is a classic example of *cucina povera*. Both potatoes and pasta are relatively cheap and rich in energy-giving carbohydrates, making this an ideal dish for those who work the land. It's even more delicious if you include chicken joints to create a *brodo*. If you do, remove the chicken before eating the soup and serve it as the *secondo*.

400g (14oz) potatoes suitable for boiling
Two or three splashes of extra-virgin olive oil
One medium-sized golden onion, finely chopped
One celery stick and leaves, finely chopped
Four skinless chicken thighs (optional)
One garlic clove, finely chopped
Handful of fresh flat-leaf parsley, finely chopped
Crushed dried red chilli (optional)
200ml (7fl oz) conserved tomato sauce (see page 263) or 200g
    (7oz) fresh plum tomatoes, skinned and chopped
Fine sea salt
400g (14oz) small pasta shapes or spaghetti snapped into pieces
    3cm (1in) long
Freshly grated Parmigiano-Reggiano or Pecorino Romano, to serve

Peel the potatoes and cut them into 1cm (½in) dice.

Heat the olive oil in a pan, and gently fry the potatoes, onion and celery together for a few minutes, until the onion is translucent.

Add the chicken thighs, if using, and cook for a minute or two until they are browned on all sides.

Add the garlic, parsley and dried chilli (if using) and cook for one minute more, stirring frequently and ensuring the garlic does not burn.

Add the tomato sauce or tomatoes to the pan along with a couple of good pinches of salt, cover the pan with a lid, and cook gently for around fifteen minutes, stirring frequently.

Next, add around 1 litre (1¾ pints) of cold water to the pan. Return to the boil, and, when the water is bubbling, add the pasta and cook for a further eight to ten minutes, or until the pasta is al dente.

Remove the chicken pieces to a warm plate, to eat after the soup.

Serve the soup immediately, sprinkled with grated *Parmiggiano-Reggiano* or *Pecorino Romano* if desired, or an extra splash of olive oil and crushed chilli.

Serves four.

Patate, mozzarella e prosciutto al forno –
Potato, mozzarella and ham bake

This is traditionally served as a *primo*, but is so rich that it makes an excellent main course, served with a crispy leaf salad. Be sure to use *fiordilatte* mozzarella made from cow's milk instead of buffalo milk, as it is drier and more suitable for cooking.

Slick of extra-virgin olive oil
1kg (2lb 3oz) potatoes suitable for boiling
Two large, fresh organic eggs
200g (7oz) Parmigiano Reggiano or Pecorino Romano, freshly grated
Fine sea salt
200g (7oz) fiordilatte mozzarella, thinly sliced
About six slices of prosciutto crudo such as Parma ham, or cooked ham, if preferred
100g (3½oz) fresh breadcrumbs

Preheat the oven to around 200°C/400°F/Gas Mark 6, and lightly oil a shallow 30 by 25cm (12 by 10in) baking dish.

Scrub the potatoes clean, place them in a pan of well-salted cold water, and bring to the boil.

Boil the potatoes for around twenty minutes, or until the centres are tender when tested with the point of a sharp knife.

When the potatoes are cool enough to handle, remove and discard the skins. Press the potatoes through a potato ricer into a large bowl, or mash thoroughly.

Beat the eggs in a bowl and add to the potatoes along with the grated cheese and a few good pinches of salt, to taste. Mix thoroughly.

Spread half the potato mixture onto the base of the oiled baking dish. Then place the mozzarella slices on top of this, in a single layer. Next lay the prosciutto slices on top of the mozzarella. Then spread the remaining half of the potato mixture on top of the prosciutto. Sprinkle the breadcrumbs over the surface of the potato bake.

Bake in the oven for around fifteen minutes then lower the heat to 180°C/350°F/Gas Mark 4, and cook for a further thirty minutes, or until the bake is golden on top.

Serves four to six.

Patate al forno – Oven-baked potatoes

This is a simple way to prepare a large amount of potatoes with a delicious meltedness – an ideal dinner-party dish.

1kg (2lb 3oz) potatoes suitable for oven baking
Plenty of extra-virgin olive oil
Few sprigs of fresh rosemary
Few cloves of garlic, still in their skins
Fine sea salt

Preheat the oven to 200°C/400°F/Gas Mark 6.

Leave the skins on the potatoes or peel them then chop into evenly sized pieces. Oil a shallow but roomy baking dish, and place the potatoes in it.

Squash the rosemary sprigs a little to bruise them, and squash the unpeeled garlic cloves against the side of a knife blade, so the flesh emerges in parts. Add the rosemary and garlic to the potatoes, and sprinkle with plenty of sea salt.

Pour a few good splashes of extra-virgin olive oil over the potatoes and stir well, ensuring the rosemary and garlic are evenly distributed among the potatoes and all the potatoes are coated in oil.

Place in the oven for around forty-five minutes or until the potatoes are soft to the blade of a sharp knife – stir them every ten minutes or so while they are cooking to ensure they cook evenly. Serve hot.

Serves six.

Forty Days in the Sun

'I've found some *amarene*.'

Few things I have said while sitting in a Campomelano kitchen have caused such a stir as my revelation that I'd managed to procure some *amarena* cherries.

I'd left it late in the season, people warned me, probably too late, and the pickings had been particularly poor due to the unusually hot weather, and those damnable birds.

But after months of hearing *amarene* talked about with almost mystical reverence, I was desperate to secure some. Little did I imagine that it would take two weeks of polite inquiries, followed by fruitless foraging attempts in the wild and, finally, more than a bit of blatant begging, to get my hands on a few kilos of the things.

I didn't truly appreciate how prized these sour cherries are around here until I returned from several *amarena* quests empty-handed. Because usually when it comes to acquiring food in Campodimele, the problem is quite the opposite. It's impossible to step over your doorstep here and return without a handful of new-laid eggs gifted to you by a friend you bumped into at the hen houses, or fresh salad leaves offered by a stranger who called you over to comment on the beautiful sunset and snapped you a lettuce from his *orto* as you chatted. I think it may in fact be illegal to allow someone to leave your house without shoving a few tomatoes into their pockets, or half a loaf of home-baked bread. Attempts to refuse such generosity are, I have always found, pointless, and, as one good friend advised, '*Chi non accetta, non merita!*' – 'She who does not accept, is not deserving.'

So I was astonished to discover that no amount of time, effort and money looked likely to procure me a few kilos of *amarena* cherries, which grow well in the high, cool spring and early summer climes of Campodimele, but are difficult to come by in markets and shops.

'These are definitely our last lot,' apologized a neighbour who has her own *amarena* trees. 'I bought these from a *contadina* – but I can't remember her name,' said another whom I chanced upon making jam outside her home. 'If you find any, we'll take 10 kilos – or more, if they have them,' begged a friend.

That's not to say the generosity had dried up – people offered me jars of their *amarena* jam, crusty *amarena* tarts, and my friend Gaetano treated me to a spoonful of his *amarene* preserved in their own syrup, splashed over ice cream. 'Not everyone who comes to lunch at my house gets the *amarene*,' he informed me solemnly. But nobody seemed willing to tell me where they had sourced the raw fruit.

So it was with more than a little disbelief that I finally got my hands on 6 kilos of *amarene*. Imagine the smallest of cherries, the darkest shade of red, the plumpest flesh. Bite into them and the sour juices wither the tongue, the tiny stone mellowing it with its almondy aftertaste. It's this sourness which gives the *amarena* its name, *amaro* being Italian for 'sour', and it is this sourness which is prized. It renders the *amarene* unpalatable in their raw state, but, mixed with the sweetness of sugar for jam or syrup, it offers the most moreish *agrodolce*, or sweet-sour, experience.

Delicious and desired as *amarene* are, there is one aspect of them which is less than likeable – their stones. Because *amarene* are around half the size of most cherries, perhaps even smaller, there are at least twice as many stones to remove per kilo before they are cooked. This is not a job for one person.

And so it is that we gather under the pergola: Amalia, Assunta, Pasqualina and me, stoning the precious *amarene*. We rinse handful after handful of fruit in a huge blue tub under the outdoor tap, decant it into smaller bowls set out on the picnic table and settle down for the afternoon, because the task ahead will take up the rest of the day.

It's painstaking work, separating the tiny stones from the juicy flesh, which will be turned into jam. It would be so much easier to walk into a shop and buy the jam, but '*i conservanti!*' exclaims Assunta at the mention of commercially produced stuff, 'the preservatives!' '*Meglio così*,' she says, 'better this way' – and it is, and not just because this *amarena* jam will be free of chemicals.

There is something timeless and beautiful about this afternoon under the pergola. The sun shafts through the vine leaves, casting the grape bunches as monstrous shadows on the stone walls of Amalia's home. Her husband, Pasquale, was born in this house, which is built above the outer edge of the village walls. No doubt his mother sat in this very spot on many afternoons, stoning *amarene* for jam, shelling borlotti beans for dinner, slicing vegetables for minestrone.

Because these are the jobs that fall to the women. 'The men do the heavy work, the women the lighter work at home,' explains Amalia. Like so many people in Campodimele, she and Pasquale still retain a *terreno*, in ages gone by the only source of food and income for millions of *contadini* across Italy. Today many who have office jobs and careers outside the village choose to continue the tradition of the *terreno*. As in the past, it is often – though not always – the men who sow, tend and harvest the land while the women process the fruits of their labours at home.

Like so much of the work involved in preserving foods, this is methodical, repetitive. It could be boring, but it isn't. It's a pleasure, fun, and I understand that afternoons like this are an integral part of the social fabric of Campodimele. They are an excuse for women to gather, chat and laugh about life, food, family. After seven decades of stoning *amarene*, Assunta still thinks a day like today is the perfect excuse to squirt the juicy red fruit at our faces, to slather her stained fingers across our cheeks. This easy sociability beneath sun-spangled pergolas can be seen throughout the village in the spring and summer months; these are moments in which the womenfolk can be still, but remain productive, because, as they will tell you, *'in campagna, c'è sempre da fare'* – in the countryside, there is always something to do.

We are nearly done. Just a kilo or so of *amarene* remains, and these last are not to be stoned. Instead they'll be used to make the renowned *amarene in sciroppo*, perhaps the most prized *amarena* product in these parts. Pasqualina piles a mountain of fruit into a large glass jar then pours caster sugar straight from the box on top of them. The snow-white sugar cascades like an avalanche, over, under, between the *amarene*. Pasqualina fixes a tight lid on the jar and tells me to leave it in a sunny spot for forty days, tipping it upside down for a moment every day. The heat of the Italian sun will meld the juice of the fruit and the sugar into a delicious syrup, which will preserve the fruit to provide a splash of summer in winter.

But not all the *amarene* are gone, I realize, as a squirt of dark juice splashes across my cheek. Assunta's laughter and her dancing black eyes give her away. These are good *amarene*, juicy, she says mischievously: 'Where did you find them this late in the season?'

How to respond? I procured them via a local businessman, who knows a *contadina*, who sometimes sells a crate or two of *amarene*. He couldn't tell me her name, or where she lives, and didn't have her phone number handy – but he would ring her for me, if I was really stuck. So it was that twenty-four hours afterwards he'd found me 6 kilos – but still couldn't remember the old lady's name. And no, there weren't any more to be had. Not until next year.

I shrugged, as a dozen villagers had shrugged at me on my *amarena* quest, and gave Assunta a puzzled smile. 'I'm afraid I can't say. They come from a *contadina*. But I've no idea of her name. And I'm afraid they're the very last of the year.'

Marmellata di amarene – Amarena jam

This recipe uses around a quarter of the sugar many British jam-makers would use for a traditional fruit conserve. However, the more sugar you use, the more you mask the sourness of the *amarena*, and it is the *agrodolce* balance that makes this jam so sought after. A lower sugar content means lower conservation quality, though, so this jam should be eaten sooner rather than later – not that it is likely to last long once you've tried it!

1 kg (2lb 3oz) amarene
Between 250g and 500g (9oz and 1lb 2oz) caster sugar, accord-
*   ing to taste*
Two 500ml (1 pint) glass jars with screw tops

Place a saucer in your freezer.

To sterilize glass jars, first wash them in hot soapy water, ensuring they are scrupulously cleaned. Preheat the oven to 160°C/320°F/Gas Mark 3, place the jars upright on an oven tray then place them in the oven for half an hour or so until they are thoroughly dry. Do the same with the lids, but remove them from the oven the moment they are dry, to avoid warping.

Stone the *amarene*, place them in a large pan, and bring the fruit to the boil, stirring often to prevent sticking.

Allow the cherries to boil for around a minute then scatter the sugar over the fruit, stirring constantly, and bring the jam mixture back to the boil, boiling for three to four minutes.

To test if the jam is at setting point, pour a small amount onto the freezer-chilled saucer and tilt the saucer – if the jam sticks to the saucer and ripples, it is ready. If it runs, boil the jam for another minute then test it on the saucer again – continue doing this until it is ready.

Once the jam is ready, pour it into the sterilized glass jars, seal with the screw lids, and turn the jars upside down for half an hour. Store in a cool place, away from direct light.

Makes about two 500ml (1 pint) jars of jam.

Crostata all'amarena — Amarena-jam tart

Shortcrust pastry in Campodimele is traditionally made with *strutto*, lard from the pig which most households once kept to provide prosciutto, *pancetta* and *salsicce*. If you are unable to find pig's lard, use butter.

You will need a shallow tart tin, measuring around 27 centimetres (11 inches) in diameter, for this recipe.

500g (1lb 2oz) '00' Doppio Zero flour or plain flour
120g (4oz) strutto or butter — at room temperature and chopped into small pieces
120g (4oz) caster sugar
½ tsp bicarbonate of soda
Three medium-sized fresh organic eggs, beaten
Grated rind of a small lemon — no pith — or phial of lemon oil
250g (9oz) amarena jam, made according to the recipe on page 188, or other jam if you prefer

If using plain flour, sieve it into a large bowl; if using '00', there is no need to sieve it.

Add the *strutto* or the butter, and, using your fingertips, gently rub it into the flour until the mixture resembles breadcrumbs — as you work, scoop up the mixture and raise it high above the bowl before dropping the crumbs back into the bowl — this will help incorporate air into the pastry, making it lighter.

Add the sugar and bicarbonate of soda, and mix well to ensure it is evenly distributed. Make a well in the centre of the mixture, and pour in the beaten eggs, reserving a little to use for glazing the tart later. Add the lemon rind or oil to the egg in the flour well.

Use a fork to mix the flour into the eggs by gradually drawing the inner edges of the flour well into the egg mixture. As the mixture thickens, use your hands to draw it together, until you have a smooth ball of dough. Wrap in cling film, and leave in the fridge to rest for half an hour.

Butter the tart tin.

When the dough is rested, lightly flour your rolling pin and a large, clear work surface. Roll out the pastry – work gently, rolling out from the centre of the dough towards the outer edges and flipping it over occasionally, reflouring the work surface and the pin as you go.

When you have a pastry disc of around 35cm (14in) in diameter, use it to line the buttered tart tin.

Use a knife to cut away the overhanging edges of pastry, reserving the offcuts to make the *strisciarelle*.

Preheat the oven to 160°C/320°F/Gas Mark 3.

Spread the jam over the base of the tart.

Now make the *strisciarelle*. Roll out the offcuts into a rectangle about 35cm (14in) in length, and cut into six ribbons around 1cm (½in) wide.

Use half of the remaining beaten egg to glaze the circumference of the pastry case then arrange the *strisciarelle* over the surface of the jam in a lattice effect – pressing the edges of the ribbons well down onto the crust. Use the remaining half of the egg to glaze the *strisciarelle*.

Cook in the oven for around half an hour – or until the pastry is golden.

Allow to cool in the tin, and serve at room temperature.

Serves eight to ten.

Amarene in sciroppo — Amarene in their own syrup

These *amarene* are bottled in glass and dressed with sugar before being left in the sun for forty days. The cherries marinate in their own juices and the sugar, resulting in a delicious syrup sauce.

1kg (2lb 3oz) amarene, stones still in
250g (9oz) caster sugar

Choose a glass jar large enough to hold all the *amarene* and the sugar, and sterilize it (see page 188).

Once the jar is sterilized, allow it to cool, then pile the *amarene* into it.

Next pour the sugar into the jar so that it cascades down and around the *amarene*. Put the lid on the jar and leave it in a place where it will receive direct sunlight for forty days.

Every day tip the jar upside down for a moment to redistribute the sugar syrup before turning it the right way up again – but do not open it.

After forty days the *amarene* should be ready to eat – they are delicious spooned over rich vanilla ice cream or stirred into sparkling mineral water and served as a drink.

Heavenly Nightshade

First find your stone; heavy but compact is the key. Next scrub off any dirt; not a speck of soil can remain. Then take a large pan, one you won't need for a day or two, and ensure the stone fits inside. Now the preserving can begin.

In Campodimele the food chain so often starts in the *orto*. Usually it's a question of snapping fruit from the plants, digging vegetables from the ground.

But now that Mafalda's garden is aglut with aubergines, she wants to save them by preserving them in oil. So her trip to the *orto* begins with the selection of a suitable stone.

Aubergines are a member of the nightshade family of fruits, a name that perfectly evokes the purply-black depths of their skins, and while their creamy flesh is a versatile base for any number of dishes, it often contains bitter juices. When aubergines first reached Italy from Africa in the fourteenth century, their bitterness was believed capable of causing craziness in those who consumed them, hence the Italian name for them: *melanzana*, derived from *mela insana*, 'mad apple'. But the Italians were not about to let such a concern get in the way of a good meal and overcame this fear to make aubergines into a mainstay of their cuisine.

Mafalda has the steady gaze of wisdom which you see in so many eyes here. It's a way of looking at the world that comes from understanding life's fundamental truths, the cycle of Nature. I can't believe she adheres to the superstition that the bitter juices in her aubergines will send her mad. But they could spoil the taste of this glut, hence the stone.

Mafalda grows the *melanzana lunga* variety, long aubergines, which are like thin curved truncheons topped with fairy-caps of papery green leaves. These are more suited to preserving than their shorter, plumper cousin, *melanzana comune*, which is the best for frying in olive oil, and *melanzana rotonda*, a johnny-come-lately whose round form is convenient for stuffing, but which seems to be regarded round here as a monster of modern bioengineering.

Mafalda welcomes me into the cool of her home one searing July afternoon and shows me how she has peeled the aubergines and sliced their flesh into long matchsticks before sprinkling them with sea salt and placing them in an aluminium pan. An old lid rests directly on the fruit, weighted down by the chalky rock she has lugged in from the garden. Just an hour into the process, the extracting qualities of the salt combined with the pressure of the stone are forcing the juices from the aubergines up the sides of the pan, marooning the rock in a pool of dark red liquid. Mafalda tips the juice out of the pan and tells me the aubergines need a minimum of twenty-four hours *sotto peso*, 'under weight', so suggests I return tomorrow.

Mafalda's home is *giù*, 'down' in the lower fraction of Campodimele known as Taverna, set back from the main road amid fruit trees and her family's *orto*.

Over espresso the following afternoon, she tells me that the airy stone house is seventy years old and that she was born there sixty-seven years ago. To raise the money needed to build the family home, *Nonno* Gaetano, her grandfather, like so many of his fellow Campomelani, migrated for a while to Toronto to work on the construction of *Il Track*, the railway infrastructure. Before he headed off to the other side of the world, his wife, *Nonna* Maria, taught him to read and write so that he could send love letters home to her. While he worked and sent money back, *Nonna* Maria oversaw the building of the house. Mafalda remembers watching her *nonna* preserving summer fruits and vegetables right here, where Mafalda is now sitting.

We tip the rock and the juices out of the pan and remove what remains of the aubergines. The matchsticks are shrunken and shrivelled, and there is an astonishingly small volume of them, considering the huge pile Mafalda put into the pan yesterday. But then this fruit is around 90 per cent water, which the stone has squeezed out.

Mafalda boils up a pan of white-wine vinegar and water and sploshes the aubergines into it to boil for a few minutes. Meanwhile, she chops the *condimenti*: parsley, garlic, chilli, oregano. After a few minutes' boiling, she drains the blanched aubergines onto her draining board amid a cloud of vinegary vapour. Once they have cooled, she squeezes the remaining liquid out of them and mixes them with the *condimenti* and some extra-virgin olive oil. Finally she spoons the mixture into jars, tops them up with oil and screws the lids on tight. *Fatto!* Done!

The aubergines can be eaten straightaway, but this is summer, the season of plenty, and the fresh fruits are in rich supply, ready to be stuffed and baked and served hot, or simmered into vegetable stews. And the point of preserving is not to eat now, but to eat later, to stock up the *cantina* for the winter. Safe under their protective covering of oil, these *melanzane* should be good for a year or so, a nutritious *contorno* for winter dinners, an instant antipasto on a hectic day.

Mafalda and her daughter-in-law, Lucia, taste-test the *melanzane* and agree that this year they are stronger than usual on the vinegar.

They have a spongy texture in the mouth, the mix of condiments a foil to their creamy blandness. But no, they are not bitter. The stone will be lugged back into the *orto* later today, having performed its task. No madness here. Just the wisdom of a life lived close to Nature, in sway with the rhythms of the land.

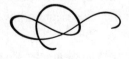

Melanzane, peperoni e cipolle al basilico —
Aubergines with red peppers, onions and basil

Two splashes of extra-virgin olive oil
Two large red peppers, deseeded and cut into slices
Two medium-sized golden onions, finely sliced into rounds
Two large aubergines
Two cloves of garlic, peeled and squashed by the side of a knife
    (optional)
Handful of fresh flat-leaf parsley, chopped (optional)
250ml (½ pint) conserved tomato sauce (see page 263) or six
    plum tomatoes, skinned and deseeded
Pinch of crushed dried red chilli (optional)
Lots of fresh basil

Heat the oil in a deep frying pan, add the pepper and onions, and cook over a medium heat for around ten minutes, making sure they do not colour.

Meanwhile, cut the aubergines into quarters lengthways then cut each quarter into thin strips.

Lower the heat in the pan. Add the aubergines, garlic and parsley, if using. Fry gently for ten minutes, stirring frequently to ensure the onions and garlic do not burn.

Add the tomato sauce or tomatoes and allow the vegetables to cook for a further five minutes or so. Add the chilli, if using.

Remove from the heat and stir in the basil. Serve with lots of fresh, crusty bread.

Serves four to six.

Melanzane con peperoni e patate –
Aubergines with red peppers and potatoes

This is a substantial one-pot main course which my friend 'Pina showed me how to make. Her recommendation to eat it cold, the next day of a hot summer, along with lots of fresh crusty bread, is one I agree with.

Modern farming has seen the development of varieties of aubergines whose bitter juices are minimal and organic aubergines often contain less water than non-organic ones. If you can procure these, do – if not, remove the juices by cutting the aubergines into slices or chunks, scattering with salt and placing in a colander covered by a sturdy plate, weighed down with heavy tins of food. Rinse off the salt and pat dry with kitchen paper. For the recipe below, an hour *sotto peso* like this should be enough – when preserving aubergines in oil, however, they need twenty-four hours under weight, to extract almost all their moisture.

Two large aubergines – the short, plump ones if possible
Few splashes of extra-virgin olive oil
One large red pepper, deseeded and cut into large slices
One large golden onion, roughly chopped
Two cloves of garlic, finely chopped
500ml (1 pint) conserved tomato sauce (see page 263)
Dried oregano
Four large, waxy potatoes, cut into even-sized chunks
Fine sea salt
Handful of fresh flat-leaf parsley, roughly chopped

Slice the aubergines lengthways, and cut each half into around six pieces. If necessary, extract the juices according to the instructions on the previous page.

Next, heat the olive oil in a large, deep pan, and gently fry the sliced pepper and chopped onion for a few minutes. Add the chopped garlic and fry for a further minute. Then add the aubergines, stir well, and fry for a minute or two more.

Add the tomato sauce or tomatoes along with a few pinches of dried oregano, bring the contents of the pan to the boil, and allow to simmer for ten minutes.

Then add the potato chunks along with a few good pinches of salt, to taste, and simmer gently until the potato centres are tender to the point of a sharp knife.

Serve sprinkled with chopped fresh parsley, or lots of fresh basil if you prefer, and lots of crusty bread.

Serves four.

Melanzane ripiene al forno – Stuffed, baked aubergines

These aubergine halves look wonderful and are as delicious cold as they are hot – a perfect side dish or vegetarian main course which can be made in advance. Try to use aubergines which don't need their juices extracted (see page 198).

Four medium-sized aubergines
Six ripe plum tomatoes, skinned, deseeded and chopped
Handful of fresh flat-leaf parsley, chopped
Fine sea salt
Two cloves of garlic, finely chopped
Handful of basil leaves, torn, plus extra to serve
Handful of black olives, stoned and halved
Extra-virgin olive oil

Preheat the oven to 200°C/400°F/Gas Mark 6.

Slice the aubergines in half lengthways. Using a sharp knife, make diagonal incisions from left to right into the flesh of each aubergine half – you need to cut almost down to the skin, but make sure not to puncture it. Then make diagonal incisions from right to left, to create a lattice effect.

In a bowl, mix together the tomatoes, parsley, two or three good pinches of salt, the garlic, basil and olives then add a splash of olive oil and mix thoroughly.

Spoon the tomato, olive and herb mixture over the aubergines, trying to persuade some of the sauce into the incisions in the flesh as you do so.

Lay the aubergine halves in a shallow baking dish and pour olive oil around them to the depth of around 1 cm (½in).

Place the dish in the oven for around forty-five minutes, until the aubergine flesh is soft through.

Remove the dish from the oven, sprinkle fresh basil over the aubergines, and allow them to rest for about fifteen minutes before serving.

Serves four as a main course, eight as a side dish.

Melanzane alla parmigiana –
Aubergine and Parmesan layers

These oven-baked aubergines in Parmesan and tomato
sauce are another recipe which has become widely used
here in the past fifty years, as better transport links have
made *Parmigiano-Reggiano*, the famous northern Italian hard
cow's milk cheese, more easily available. But the recipe also
works very well with *Pecorino Romano*, the matured sheep's
cheese that is more traditional to Campodimele – though
most people seem to use the new arrival in my experience!
Be sure to choose *fiordilatte* mozzarella, which is more
suited to baking than *mozzarella di bufala*. You may need to
extract the juices from the aubergines an hour in advance.

Four large aubergines, sliced into rounds, juices extracted
    if necessary (see page 198)
Handful of '00' Doppio Zero flour or plain flour
Four good splashes of extra-virgin olive oil
400g (14oz) fiordilatte mozzarella
One medium-sized golden onion, finely chopped
500ml (1 pint) conserved tomato sauce (see page 263)
Fine sea salt
Good handful of fresh basil leaves, torn
200g (7oz) chunk of Parmigiano-Reggiano or Pecorino Romano,
    freshly grated

Preheat the oven to 180°C/350°F/Gas Mark 4.

Dust the aubergine slices with flour, heat the oil in a
large frying pan, and fry them over a medium heat quickly,

until they are golden on both sides. Remove to a plate covered with kitchen paper, and pat them to remove all excess oil.

Now cut the the mozzarella into fine slices.

To make the tomato sauce, gently fry the onion in olive oil for around five minutes then add the tomato conserve and a good pinch of salt. Remove from the heat and stir in the fresh basil.

In a shallow baking dish, first slick a thin layer of tomato sauce and then a layer of aubergines, followed by a layer of grated Parmesan and a layer of mozzarella. Cover with more tomato sauce then repeat the layers until you have used up all the aubergines. Finish with a layer of tomato sauce, topped by a few slices of mozzarella, reserving a little of the Parmesan to scatter over the top later.

Bake in the oven for thirty minutes then sprinkle with the remaining Parmesan and bake for ten more minutes until the cheese is golden. Rest for around fifteen minutes before serving.

Serves four to six.

Melanzane sott'olio – Aubergines preserved in oil

Aubergines are about 90 per cent water, and since the juices must be thoroughly extracted the day before preserving, a large quantity of these fruits will produce a surprisingly small quantity of preserves – but a little bit of *melanzane sott'olio* goes a long way on the plate, so don't be too disappointed!

5kg (11lb) aubergines – try to get the long, thin variety
Fine sea salt
1 litre (2 pints) white-wine vinegar
Four cloves of garlic, finely chopped
Handful of fresh flat-leaf parsley, finely chopped
Good sprinkling of dried red chilli or fresh, if you prefer
Good sprinkling of dried oregano
1 litre (2 pints) or so extra-virgin olive oil
Around three 350ml (12fl oz) glass jars with airtight lids,
    sterilized (see page 188)

Peel the aubergines, discarding the skins, and slice the flesh into thin matchsticks. Sprinkle plenty of fine sea salt over them, and follow the instructions on page 198 to extract the juices. Leave them *sotto peso* for twenty-four hours, pouring away the juices every so often to ensure the aubergines are not resting in them.

Once the juices have been extracted from the aubergine matchsticks, boil about 1 litre (2 pints) of water and 1 litre (2 pints) of white-wine vinegar in a large pan. Boil the aubergine in this liquid for around five minutes.

Drain the aubergines and lay out to cool on a flat, clean surface. Once they have cooled, squeeze them between your palms a handful at a time to extract the cooking liquid – a large-bellied potato ricer can be effective for extracting water this way. Use a clean tea towel or kitchen paper to pat off any excess liquid.

Place the aubergines in a bowl and mix in the garlic, parsley, chilli and oregano, adding a pinch or two of fine sea salt.

Pour a small amount of olive oil into each sterilized glass jar. Then pile the dressed aubergines into the jars, to within 2cm (1in) of the neck. Fill the jar with olive oil, tilting the jar as you do so to eliminate air pockets. Make sure the aubergines are fully covered before putting the lid in place.

Leave the flavours to meld for at least four weeks. The aubergines should keep for up to a year in a cool, dark place. Once opened, they should be kept in the fridge and eaten quickly – after removing part of the contents of a jar, top up with olive oil to ensure the fruits remain covered.

Makes roughly three 350ml (12fl oz) jars.

AUGUST

Coming Around Again

How to work the land in this heat? How to suffer the scorch on the skin, the blinding light in the eyes? These August days unfurl in extremes: explosive dawns, stifling noons, sunsets which flame like the forest fires that are sparking on the parched earth. These are days made for slipping down the mountain to catch the coastal breeze or sheltering behind shuttered windows at home. But the growing season is at its peak, the *orto* is overflowing with ripeness, and wherever you look, people are in the fields.

It's 4.00 on a Friday afternoon in Taverna. You can hear the whine of a passing scooter on the road that winds through the lower village, and the mechanical buzz of a combine harvester as it devours a field of wheat. But it's a more primitive, rhythmical sound that catches my ears as I enter Ricardo's *orto*.

The *livio* is the kind of tool you would expect to see in a medieval book of hours: two long, thin, smooth branches attached to each other by a strip of leather nailed into one end of each branch. Ricardo is using the *livio* to beat *cicerchie*, the tiny pulses particular to Campodimele, in just the way that generations of his ancestors used it before him. He casts me a grin, then screws his currant-brown eyes up to glance at the sun, as if in tacit acknowledgement of the impossibility of the heat, the necessity of the day on the land.

The harvest began a week ago, as the pointed green leaves of the *cicerchie* withered to yellow straggles in the sun, the pods shrivelling against the plump pulses within.

Ricardo cut down the plants seven days ago, gathering them into bundles and leaving them to dry in the field. Now they look like clusters of tumbleweed, the pod-skins brittled by the heat.

Ricardo strews the plants onto a plastic groundsheet and, holding one branch of the *livio* with both hands, flips the second branch up and back above his head, then flicks it forward to bring it thrashing down. Shards of dried pod splatter upwards against the sunlight then shower to the ground, to be thrashed again and again. Eventually the pods lie shattered, spilling their pulses. Ricardo drops his *livio* and piles the pieces into a *setaccio*, a large sieve, shimmying it to and fro so that the *cicerchie* dribble through the holes, small and cream-coloured and angular. So much work to harvest such a tiny pulse, but, as Ricardo says, *cicerchie* have a flavour all their own.

I'd never tasted *cicerchie*, never heard of them before I came here, but whenever I mention to people from the surrounding towns and villages that I live in Campodimele, they instantly start talking about *cicerchie*, because the village is as famous for this pulse as it is for its sobriquet of '*Il Paese della Longevità*'. *Cicerchie* are served in *zuppa della nonna*, 'grandmother's soup', or boiled then splashed with olive oil and mixed with squashed garlic cloves and fragments of hot chilli pepper. Or they are cooked by a wood fire in a *pignatta*, the terracotta, two-handled jug particular to this area, the wood-smoke permeating the pulses. Perhaps together with a little *baccalà*, dried salt cod, or just a garlic clove or two. The flavour of the *cicerchie* is not like anything I have encountered before – there is a certain earthiness, a certain mustiness, a firm but smooth texture in the mouth. As Ricardo says, the flavour is unique.

But it's not just the taste of the *cicerchie* that has led to them featuring in the Campomelano diet despite the immense amount of work they take to harvest. In the past they have proved a vital source of sustenance. Along with borlotti beans, *fagioli*, broad beans and other pulses, they were part of *la carne dei poveri*. Added to this, they were an ideal crop for this mountainous terrain.

'*Cicerchie* will grow anywhere,' says Aguillino di Fonzo as we drink coffee in Maurizio's bar by the roadside in Taverna. 'Even in this *terra povera*.' Aguillino casts a hand upwards in a gesture encompassing the poor earth of Campodimele. I have never thought of the land around here in these terms before – the food culture is so rich, the fields so abundant with vegetables and fruit, mountain goats and game. But Aguillino's words bring home to me that these flat fields of wheat, these neatly stepped terraces of green, these animal-fertilized *orti* have been hard-hewn from the mountains, with their steep contours and stony soil which struggles to retain the sparse summer rainfall.

The hardy nature of *cicerchie* was to prove vital during and after World War II, when much of the farmland in Italy went to waste because there were no men to tend it.

'There was nothing to eat then,' says Aguillino, who grew up in Campodimele and remembers *cicerchie* as a significant part of his childhood diet. 'And you could rely on *cicerchie* to grow in even the poor ground, so that's what people grew.'

But as Italy embraced the industrial age and living standards improved, *cicerchie* were found on fewer and fewer plates, associated as they were with the difficult days after the war. In the past few years, however, people have returned to growing them more and more. In fact right now, the village can't get enough of this little pulse.

Tomorrow, Campodimele will host the *Sagra delle Cicerchie* – the Feast of the *Cicerchie*, staged just as the harvest is underway.

I had imagined that this *sagra* would be older than memory, its roots in an act of religious thanksgiving, but that's not the case. It began in 1991 as an initiative to bring more visitors to the village. Aguillino and a number of friends on the Pro Loco Campodimele, the development agency, decided that the *cicerchie*, grown in few other parts of Italy, was the perfect vehicle to attract more people to their area. Naturally, the decision was made around the kitchen table. 'We met for dinner at my house to discuss it,' recalls Aguillino. 'We ate *cicerchie* – and agreed that this was something special the village should make more of.'

The initiative worked. Today more than fifteen different types of *cicerchie* are being grown in Campodimele as part of a study in conjunction with the University of Viterbo to identify which kind thrives best here. This is a first step to increase production as part of a plan for economic development.

From where Ricardo is thrashing the *cicerchie* you can hear the women's laughter, their voices swimming through the shimmering air. I find them beneath the trees by the house. Lucia, Maria-Civita, Rita, Immacolata and Antonella are seated around a *mallia* piled high with *cicerchie*. These are not the little sun-dried stones which Ricardo is harvesting. These *cicerchie* are twice the size, swollen after long hours of soaking in water along with a little bicarbonate of soda to persuade the softening process.

The women rake their hands through the piles of pulses in search of darkly discoloured ones, chipped ones, ones which have tiny holes in the surface, betraying the insects that have burrowed inside while the pulse was still on the plant, so ruining it. There are 65 kilos in all: 65 kilos to soak for almost forty-eight hours, to sort by hand then to set to boil so that the *sagra* can begin.

Washing the soaked *cicerchie* is the important thing, says Lucia as Rita drains the pulses yet again into the sink of the *asilo*, the communal building in Taverna where the *sagra* food is being prepared. Three changes of water at least, she adds, or you can give yourself a bad stomach. Particularly important when you are cooking for the entire village and the hordes who will flock to Taverna tonight.

Now they are bubbling in pans everywhere – in huge aluminium vats on the *asilo* stove, and over portable gas cookers set up in its reception corridor, sending the temperature spilling over on this outrageously hot August day. The *cicerchie* are being cooked by *la stessa squadra*, the same team who prepared them yesterday and who have cooked them for the past sixteen *sagre*. They chop prosciutto to add, scraping away the scum floating on the tops of the vats.

'*Ognuna di noi giudica*' – 'Every one of us judges,' they say, unfazed at the notion of preparing food for thousands of Italians, each one with the firmest of opinions on what tastes good and what doesn't. Now they collectively taste-test the *cicerchie* and agree that they are *buone*, good, ready to eat.

Such *sagre* are the quintessential Italian social gathering, I think later, as I join the queue for my tray of cooked *cicerchie*. Food, music, dancing *all' aperto*, 'in the open air.' Crowds have flocked to Campodimele from the towns and villages around to get a taste of the famous *cicerchie* and yes, they agree, they are good – soft to the bite with the sweet tang of prosciutto.

Here, tonight, as the *cicerchie* are celebrated, it's hard to believe that they once smacked of bad times, once struggled to find a place in the *orto*. It feels right to think they could aid prosperity in the years to come. Everything has its season, as I am often told here. That of the *cicerchie*, it seems, is here again.

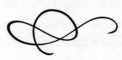

Cicerchie al prosciutto – Cicerchie with prosciutto

This simple recipe would traditionally have been served after the pasta course as a *secondo* along with a *contorno* of leafy greens or other vegetables.

The *cicerchie* must be soaked with bicarbonate of soda for at least thirty-six hours prior to cooking. If you are lucky enough to have a wood-burning stove or fire at home, use it to cook the pulses, allowing the wood-smoke to flavour them. If you are unable to find *cicerchie*, these recipes also work well with dried chickpeas, also known as garbanzo beans.

450g (1lb) dried cicerchie
Pinch of bicarbonate of soda
100g (3½oz) thick-sliced prosciutto, finely chopped
Extra-virgin olive oil
Fine sea salt

To prepare the *cicerchie*, soak them for thirty-six to forty-eight hours, along with a pinch of bicarbonate of soda to aid the softening process and speed up the cooking time. Change the soaking water three or four times, remembering to add a pinch of bicarb to every change of water. Once the *cicerchie* are ready to cook, it is essential to rinse them thoroughly – at least three further changes of water are recommended – in order to get rid of the juices that can lead to stomach upset unless washed away.

Rinse the *cicerchie* thoroughly then place them in a large pan along with enough fresh cold water to cover them by about 10cm (4in). Cover the pan and bring to the boil, skimming off any scum which rises to the surface.

Add the chopped prosciutto, reduce the heat, and simmer the *cicerchie* briskly until they are tender to the bite, removing scum as it rises to the surface. *Cicerchie* usually take around ninety minutes to cook, but this will vary depending on the size and age of your pulses.

Splash with olive oil and a little salt, if preferred.

Serves four to six.

Zuppa della nonna — Grandmother's soup

If you have some chicken stock, it will make this soup all the more delicious. If not, use vegetable stock or water.

You will need to prepare the *cicerchie* thirty-six hours in advance of making the soup.

200g (7oz) dried cicerchie
Pinch of bicarbonate of soda
Good splash of extra-virgin olive oil
One golden onion, sliced into very fine half-moons
One stick of celery, finely chopped
One clove of garlic, finely chopped
Handful of fresh flat-leaf parsley, finely chopped
250ml (½ pint) conserved tomato sauce (see page 263)
Fine sea salt
500ml (1 pint) chicken brodo (see page 59) or vegetable stock
    (optional)
200g (7oz) fresh egg tagliolini (see pages 51 and 59) or small
    pasta shapes such as snapped spaghetti or tagliatelle
Parmigiano-Reggiano or Pecorino Romano, freshly grated, to serve
    (optional)
Crushed dried red chilli (optional)

Soak the dried *cicerchie* along with the bicarbonate of soda, as described on page 214.

Rinse thoroughly in several changes of fresh cold water then place in a large pan of cold water and bring to the boil. Cover and simmer until the *cicerchie* are tender to the bite – usually around ninety minutes.

About twenty minutes before the *cicerchie* are ready to eat, heat the olive oil in a wide, deep pan, add the onion and celery, and gently fry for around ten minutes.

Add the garlic and parsley, and continue to fry for a further five minutes, stirring to ensure that the garlic does not burn.

Add the tomato sauce and three or four pinches of salt.

Once the *cicerchie* are tender, drain them and add them to the pan of tomato sauce, mixing gently to ensure each pulse is coated with the mixture.

Add the chicken *brodo* or the vegetable stock or water, depending on what you are using.

Reduce to a gentle simmer then add the pasta to the pan and continue to cook until it is al dente – perhaps a couple of minutes if using fresh *tagliolini*, or according to the instructions on the packet if using dried pasta.

Serve hot, sprinkled with freshly grated Parmesan or crushed dried chilli, if desired.

Serves four to six.

Cicerchie in pignatta con baccalà –
Cicerchie cooked in a pignatta with salt cod

When wood fires were the only heat source in the country home, the *pignatta* became the traditional way of cooking all beans and pulses. Because most homes in Campodimele still have open wood fires today, these smoke-blackened cooking jugs, made from terracotta, are still used to cook *cicerchie*. Alternatively you could easily cook this dish in a conventional oven using a terracotta casserole with a tight-fitting lid.

450g (1lb) dried cicerchie
Pinch of bicarbonate of soda
One small piece, about 125g (4oz), of dried salt cod
Two cloves of garlic, peeled and squashed by the side of a knife
Few sprigs of fresh flat-leaf parsley
Around 200ml (7fl oz) conserved tomato sauce (see page 263)

Soak the *cicerchie* in cold water for at least thirty-six hours along with the bicarbonate of soda. Then rinse thoroughly in several changes of fresh, cold water.

Soak the salt cod in a large, separate bowl of cold water for around twenty-four to thirty-six hours. Change the water frequently – several times a day if you can – in order to rid it of the salt used to preserve it.

When both the *cicerchie* and the *baccalà* are prepared, place half the *cicerchie* in the *pignatta* – or the terracotta casserole, if using – along with a clove of garlic, a few parsley sprigs and half the tomato sauce.

Next add the *baccalà*, followed by the remaining garlic, parsley, *cicerchie* and tomato sauce.

Fill the *pignatta* almost to the top with boiling water, replace the lid, and place right beside a fire for several hours, until the *cicerchie* are tender to the bite – this will take at least four hours, perhaps a little or a lot longer, depending on the age and size of your pulses and, crucially, the level of heat from your fire. So check frequently to judge progress, and to ensure there is sufficient water to cover the pulses.

If using a conventional oven, fill the casserole with water and place on the middle shelf at 180°C/350°F/Gas Mark 4 for two to four hours, until the *cicerchie* are tender to the bite.

Serve hot along with lots of fresh, crusty bread.

Serves four to six.

Cicerchie al sugo rosso – Cicerchie in red sauce

450g (1lb) dried cicerchie
Pinch of bicarbonate of soda
One large golden onion, finely chopped
One stick of celery, finely chopped
Two splashes of extra-virgin olive oil
Handful of fresh celery leaves, chopped
Large handful of fresh flat-leaf parsley, chopped
Two cloves of garlic, peeled and squashed by the side of a knife
500ml (1 pint) conserved tomato sauce (see page 263)

Soak the *cicerchie* for around thirty-six hours along with
the bicarbonate of soda as described on page 214. Rinse the
cicerchie thoroughly in several changes of cold water.

In a large, deep pan, gently fry the finely chopped onion
and celery stick in the oil for a few minutes. Add the celery
leaves, parsley and garlic, and fry for a few minutes more,
until the onion is translucent, but not coloured.

Add the drained *cicerchie* and stir to coat all the pulses
with the vegetable and herb mixture. Add 500ml (1 pint) of
cold water to the pan, stir, and bring to the boil.

Add the tomato sauce. Return to the boil.

Partially cover the pan and cook over a medium heat
until the *cicerchie* are tender to the bite, adding more water
if necessary to make sure they remain covered.

Serves four to six.

From Field to Forno

The wheat fields whisper on these August nights.

Walking by moonlight along unlit tracks, I'd swear that there are words in their sighs, an incantation in their windswept swaying. Though when we pause to catch their message, the translation escapes me still. The song of the fields rasps sharper night by night; parched by the sun, grown tall under its rays, a million wheat blades scrape and sing as one as they bend in the breeze. Snap off an ear of wheat and it feels so dry as to be dead: bullet-hard grains within their papery skins, the flower spikes like needle pricks against your hand.

We've had day after day of impossible sun; heat hazes hovering above the fields. The last storm spilt oceans of rain onto the land and split the black night with golden lightning cracks: the next can't be far away.

So it's time to harvest the wheat. To collect the grain, to wash it by hand and scatter it on the piazza to dry in the sun. Then to grind it to *farina*, fine-ground flour, and turn it into the food without which no meal in Campodimele is served: our daily bread.

Gerardo's scooter buzzes down the mountain, crackling like a cricket gone crazy. It's a journey he's making daily just now. He kick-starts his *moto* in the *centro storico* and slaloms downhill, left and right around the jay-walking hens by their ramshackle huts.

At the statue of Padre Pio the road forks – upwards to the valley-view piazza, or down to the valley floor, where Gerardo's wheat field lies. It's a 3 kilometre tumble to Taverna, a journey of leafy green tunnels where the air stays cool, of hairpin bends which slow him to the pace of a snail. A pause at the *bivio*, the junction with the mountain road, and a turn sharp right. A curve left, around the bad 90 degree bend, and Gerardo will cut the motor and stop.

'*La trebbia*,' he said last night, as he told me how he would spend this afternoon after weeks of watching his wheat, monitoring the weather, choosing the day. This word translates as 'combine harvester', but means so much more than that. '*La trebbia*' is shorthand for that moment in the agricultural calendar that is the harvesting of the wheat, followed by the hand-washing of the grain and the sun-drying of the seed. It symbolizes the satisfaction of reaping what you invested time to sow, your faith in Nature's annual gifts. But most of all it signals to Gerardo, who is now seventy-nine, his wife, Leana, and others who still grow their own wheat – even here, today, they are few – that the cupboard is full. There's enough grain in the storehouse to last the year; there will be enough bread to sate the honest hunger earned from a day working the fields.

From field to *forno*: from the field to the wood-fired oven. The whole cycle of the grain is in these words, I think, as I sit among the stubble of Maria and Michele's field on this summer's morning.

From this level, it's a gold-spun world: a vista of faded yellow wheat, yet to be culled, horizoned by the thinnest strip of gilded air. Papery red poppies and purple-blue cornflowers flutter a fare-well, and I realize that soon I'll have no more armfuls of meadow flowers to fill the terracotta *pignattas* that decorate my fireplace.

'*Cipolla selvatica*,' says Maria, as I hold up a sculptural spray-head of white-tipped flower: wild onion. When she was a girl, she tells me, children and women would come to the meadows in May and pluck these *fiori dei campi,* flowers of the fields, one by one, to stop them multiplying. The sheaves of wheat were harvested with hand-held scythes in those days, the grain sorted by hand, weeds and flowers removed as they went. It was the work of days, and the more flowers removed in May, the fewer to filter out come the harvest. Today *la trebbia* is doing all these jobs and more in the space of an hour, devouring the wheat in rhythmic beats. Up the field, down the field, up and down, now stopping where I sit. And it's done. The harvest is in. In days gone by, when the land was the *contadini*'s only form of income, this was *veramente un giorno di gioia,* nods Maria, truly a day of joy, because you knew you would have enough flour, bread and pasta in the year to come.

It's almost midday. In times gone by this was the moment when the workers would pause and shelter under trees for lunch. Lunch would be a hunk of bread, a chunk of cheese, perhaps a slice of *salsiccia sott'olio.* A tomato or two, plums, maybe an early fig. If they were working someone else's fields, the landlord might lay on the lunch, then deduct the cost from the field labourers' pay.

Those who produced enough at home would bring their own food. Perhaps a *culo del pane,* literally the bottom of the bread, the rounded end of a home-made loaf, its top sliced off, its innards pulled out and stuffed with layers of *verdure* – roasted red peppers, griddled aubergines, preserved artichokes – then the bread lid popped on again. The *culo del pane* would be made by the women last thing at night and left to rest, the oil melding the flavours of the layers, drenching the bread so it disintegrated between the teeth the next day. Drinking water would be hauled up from the wells, or perhaps there might be some red wine.

Today there's no need to remain in the fields to eat. There are two-wheeled scooters and three-wheeled Ape farm trucks and four-wheel drives to zip us home. But we mark the moment all the same by cracking open bottles of chilled Nastro Azzurro beer and drinking it from plastic picnic cups.

The piazza of the medieval *centro storico* is paved with wheat. Millions of grains scattered within the walls. This scene has been played out on this square every summer for perhaps a thousand years.

Leana scoops a handful of grain into a drum-shaped sieve and rinses cold water through it to clear the field dust. She tips it onto a plastic groundsheet and spreads the grain thinly with a brush. Leana's neighbours help her wash, clean and dry her grain, and in the days to come, she'll help them with theirs. The women will flip and turn the drying wheat under the sun by day and leave it to bathe in the moonlight by night. In the evenings they'll retire to bed and pray that it doesn't rain.

The prayers worked: the storm held off. The grain dried beneath cloudless days and starry nights. It was collected into clean sacks and stored in *magazzini*. A bagful or two at a time, as the women require it for pasta and bread, it will be transported to a local mill and ground into flour.

Once this was the moment when the villagers did pray for rain so the first batch of wheat could be ground at the *mulino del mal tempo*, the 'bad-weather mill' – a grain mill powered by water from a gulley that runs dry during hot spells, but cascades torrential in thunderstorms. Over the years, however, the weather-capricious mill fell into disuse. Today most people drive to the nearby town of Pontecorvo to mill their wheat.

But the *mulino del mal tempo* has been restored by the council of Campodimele. I've seen it come to life. One morning the summer sky awoke grey and swollen and spat spears of rain for hours. We went down to the secluded woodland where the *mulino del mal tempo* stands and watched as the watercourse leapt downhill and set the mill wheel aspin. And I remembered that even today, the simplest slice of bread only makes it to our table by the grace of forces that we can't control.

What was the moment when this bread truly began, I wonder, as Maria kneads the dough she has created from her own flour.

She's been working this *pasta* – the all-purpose word for any mix of flour and liquid – since 5.30 this morning, having risen in the first cool moments of what promises to be a scorching day.

It began last night, she tells me, when she sieved the flour to remove the *crusca*, the outer skin of the wheat grain, leaving the white powdery *grano* and its fibrous coating, the *semola*.

But in a sense, this bread began last October, when Michele scattered the wheat seeds on his fields to produce the flour his wife is handling now; or on that day when I sat in Maria and Michele's meadow and watched *la trebbia*. Though as Maria talks on, I realize it all started much longer ago than that.

'*Secoli fa*,' she says, with that dismissive back-flick of the wrist which Italians use to indicate a moment lived so long ago that we will never pin it down: centuries ago. That's when the leavening Maria uses as the raising agent in her sourdough bread was made.

This *lievito* is a family heirloom and typical of the leavenings used around here. Begun once upon a time, presumably by some female relative of Maria, this legacy has been guarded by the women of her family ever since. Perhaps it was created by Maria's *bisnonna*, her great-grandmother, or someone who lived a century or two before her. Whoever it was, they created the *lievito madre*, the 'mother leavening', by mixing flour and water and allowing it to ferment in a warm place for a few days, catching wild yeasts from the air. It is a sourdough, so *niente birra*, as they say, 'no beer' – by which they mean none of the brewer's yeast typically employed in mass-produced breads in the West today. The bubbling mass that resulted provided the leavening agent for a first batch of bread, and from that first lot of dough a small handful was reserved and used as the leavening for a second set of loaves. And from that batch another handful of uncooked dough was saved, to serve as the *lievito* for a third day of baking bread.

And so on and on, down the centuries, from *nonna*, to *figlia*, to *nipote* – grandmother to daughter to granddaughter – until here we are, wondering how many grains of flour from that original *lievito madre* will be in the bread Maria is making this morning.

Maria's house is modern, little more than twenty years old, but she is making bread the way her family have for generations. She hand-mixes the flour, water, salt and leavening in a *maniella*, a huge, deep wooden tray with handled corners. She will bake the bread in the *forno a legna* built into her chimney wall. It takes her half an hour, perhaps more, to knead the dough, and when it's done she swaddles the *maniella* in woollen blankets and leaves the dough to grow.

Pane al forno, bread baked in a wood-fired oven. These words are always spoken with a certain reverence here, even though they are used to describe the simplest of foods, because *pane al forno* is the epitome of *cibo genuino*.

Leana rises at 4.00 a.m. to bake her bread. Even in the hottest months, you can spot her walking through the village, branches piled high on her head atop a cushion of her wrapped-up cardigan, to fire up her oven. The wood of her *forno* is burned to *brace* and the loaves left to bake slowly in its heat, the slightest whiff of wood-smoke seeping into the dough.

Leana's *forno* is on the upper floor of her house, which could be almost a thousand years old. Ten centuries' worth of baking bread. Hers is densely textured brown bread beneath the brick-hard crust that contributes to Campodimele bread's renowned longevity – freshness for five, six, even seven days. Once the mainstay of *cucina povera*, bread is still served in endless ways here – even once it's gone stale. Freshly sliced, it's the accompaniment to every lunch and dinner, used to mop up spaghetti sauces and vegetable juices, what Italians call *la scarpetta*, 'the little shoe' – though nobody can tell me why. When it's a bit stale, Leana might turn it into *bruschetta* by slicing and toasting it and topping it with tomatoes, basil and olive oil; in winter, the stalest cuts will be laid in soup bowls, layered between ladlefuls of thick bean soup to create a warming *zuppa*.

'*Il pane non si butta mai via*,' says Leana, cutting me a slice. It's a simple, but now familiar, phrase which encompasses the versatility of a loaf and its significance to *cucina povera*. 'You never throw bread away.'

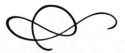

Lievito madre – Sourdough starter

Typical Campodimele bread uses a sourdough starter, harnessing the yeasts that are naturally occurring in flour and air. If you know someone who has a sourdough starter, beg, buy or borrow some – sourdoughs are often decades old, and the romance of their ancestry alone will surely add to the taste. Alternatively you can buy dried sourdough starter in good delicatessens; this should be rehydrated according to the instructions on the packet. Or you can create a family heirloom by making your own, never-ending sourdough starter.

4 tbsp strong white bread flour

Mix together a tablespoon of flour and a tablespoon of water in a large jug with a wide, open mouth. Leave to sit at room temperature, covered with a clean, damp tea towel, for forty-eight hours.

Add another tablespoon of flour and another of water, blend well into the original mix, and leave for another twenty-four hours.

Repeat this process for three or four days – eventually you should end up with a bubbling yeast mixture. If the mix goes mouldy, discard and start again.

Use a double batch of this sourdough as leavening for your first loaves of bread. Every time you make a loaf, reserve a handful of the sourdough and store it in the fridge to use as leavening for the next batch.

Pane al forno a legna –
Bread baked in a wood-fired oven

Every home here has its own bread recipe. This one makes two small, round loaves which are dense in texture and should stay fresh for several days in an airtight container. They remain delicious eaten stale, as toasted *bruschetta* or swamped in soups such as winter *minestra*.

400g (14oz) sourdough starter (see opposite)
500ml (1 pint) tepid water
400g (14oz) organic white strong bread flour
600g (1lb 5oz) organic wholemeal flour
2 tsp fine sea salt

The evening before you wish to make the bread, combine the sourdough starter with the tepid water and leave at room temperature overnight.

The next day, sieve the flour and combine it with the salt in a large bowl. Create a well in the centre of the flour.

Now pour the sourdough and water into the centre of the flour well and mix thoroughly – start by drawing the inner edges of the flour into the liquid, and continue like this until you have a smooth dough. If the dough feels a little sticky when most of the flour is combined, add a little more – you want a dough that is firm and smooth, with some elasticity in it.

When the dough is ready, turn out onto a floured work-top and begin to knead – flatten it on the floured work surface then draw the far edge up and over the dough towards you. Then lift the near edge up and over the dough away from you. Turn the dough through 90 degrees and repeat this process. Continue until you have a very smooth, elastic dough – this could easily take fifteen minutes.

Put the dough back in the bowl, cover with a clean, damp tea towel, and leave in a warm place to leaven to double its original size – this is likely to take at least three hours, but it could need longer, depending on your flour, the kitchen temperature and, I have found, the weather conditions on the day of baking! As a general rule, a young starter has slower leavening powers.

Then remove the bread and punch it to knock out some of the gas bubbles. Leave to leaven for a further hour or so in the covered bowl.

While the dough is leavening, if you are lucky enough to have a wood-fired oven, set the branches to burn so they will be reduced to charcoal by the time the bread is ready to bake – this could take up to two hours.

Alternatively, you can preheat a conventional oven to 220°C/425°F/Gas Mark 7.

Now tip the dough onto a floured work surface, cut in half, and gently shape each piece of dough into a round, low loaf. Place on a large greased baking sheet and cook in the hottest part of your oven for around forty minutes, or until the bread is golden brown on top – do not open the oven while it is cooking.

When the bread is ready remove from the oven, cool on a wire rack then store in an airtight container.

Makes two small loaves.

Bruschetta con pomodoro e basilico –
Tomato and basil bruschetta

*Half a small loaf of pane al forno which is two to three days old
or other bread suitable for toasting
Handful of fresh plum tomatoes
Handful of basil leaves, torn
Few splashes of extra-virgin olive oil
Four large cloves of peeled garlic, sliced in half and squashed by
the side of a knife
Fine sea salt*

Cut the bread into slices around 2 to 3cm (1in) thick.

Roughly chop the tomatoes and put them in a bowl with the basil, olive oil and one of the garlic cloves. Allow to marinate for around ten minutes.

Toast the bread – in a wood-fired oven, under the grill of your cooker or in a toaster.

Scrape the remaining halves of garlic across one side of each piece of toast, squeezing the juices into the bread as you go.

Top with the tomato, basil and oil mixture, and scatter over a pinch of salt, to taste. Eat immediately.

Serves four as a starter, or two as a quick lunch.

Culo del pane – *Bottom of the bread*

'*Culo*' is a colloquial, none-too-polite term for 'posterior' – the inelegance of the name belies the beauty of this deliciously sumptuous sandwich.

Half a round loaf of pane al forno or other coarse-textured bread
*   with a good, thick crust*
Selection of vegetables cooked or preserved in olive oil, such as red
*   peppers, artichokes and aubergines*
Handful of spinach leaves (optional)
Fine sea salt
Handful of fresh herbs, such as basil or oregano

Slice a curved end from the loaf, creating an offcut around 10cm (4in) deep.

Tear the bread out of the crusty shell, reserving it to use for mopping up sauces with your main meal.

Fill the hollowed-out crust with layers of vegetables which have been cooked or preserved in oil – for example, a layer of peppers, followed by one of sliced artichokes then another of aubergines. Interlayer with raw spinach leaves if you wish, and a sprinkling of salt and fresh herbs.

Wrap the entire *culo del pane* tightly in greaseproof paper or cling film then place it in the fridge, positioned so that the open end is uppermost – leave like this overnight, allowing the oil and vegetable juices to saturate the bread.

The next day, remove the *culo del pane* from the fridge, and allow it to return to room temperature before eating.

Serves one.

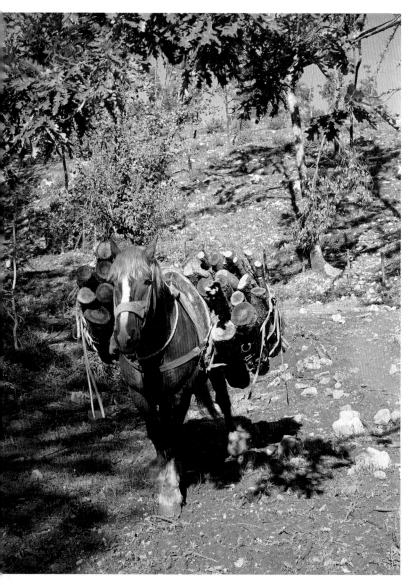

One of the horses that help to harvest the oak logs which fuel the fires and *forni* of Campodimele.

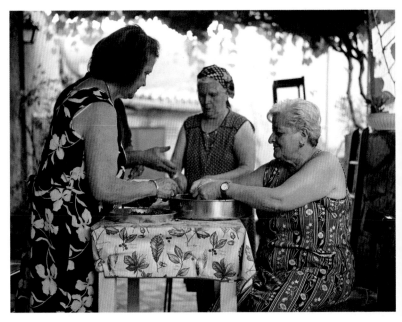

An afternoon stoning *amarena* cherries under the pergola. From left to right: Pasqualina, Assunta and Amalia.

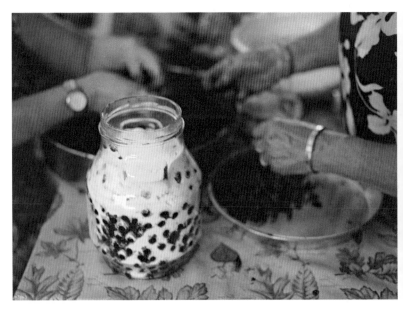

This jar of sugar and cherries will be left in the sun for forty days to make *amarena* syrup (see page 192).

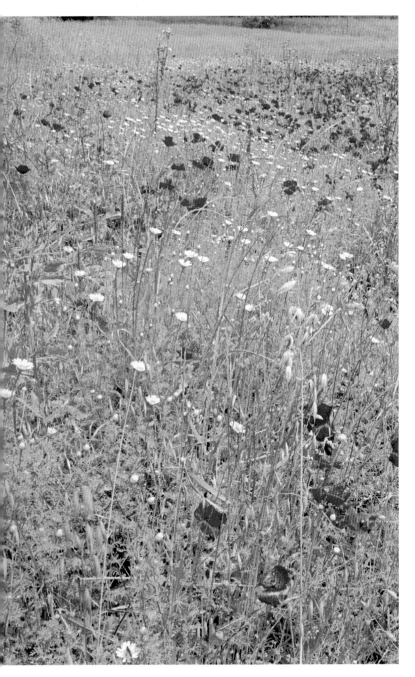

summer the meadows of Campodimele are awash with wildflowers, such as poppies.

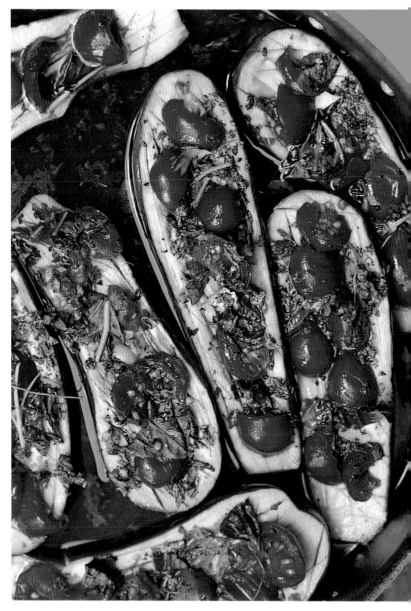

Melanzane ripiene al forno – stuffed, baked aubergines (see page 200).

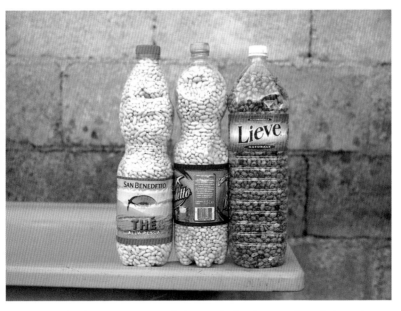

Dried *fagioli* and borlotti beans are among the beans and pulses that are traditionally key to the Campomelano *cucina*.

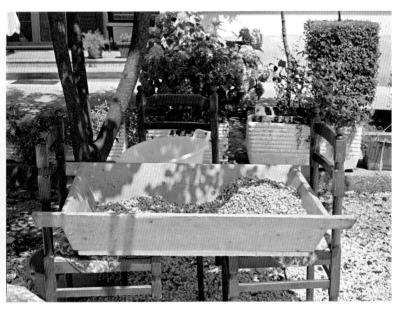

Rehydrated *ciccerchie*, the pulse particular to Campodimele, waiting to be cooked for the *Sagra delle Ciccerchie* in August.

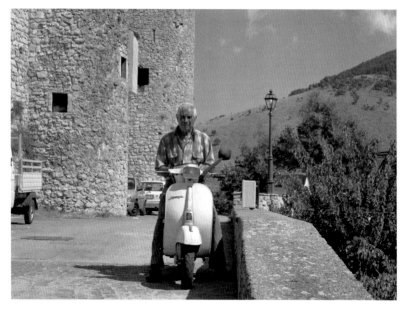

Gerardo zips up and down the squiggly mountain road on his Vespa, to monitor his wheat field on the valley floor.

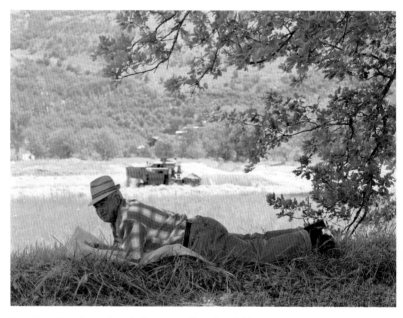

La trebbia – Gerardo watching the harvesting of his wheat field.

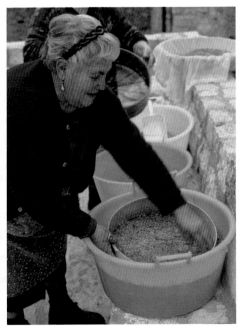

Gerardo's wife Leana washes
the wheat grain, before
scattering it in the piazza
to sun-dry.

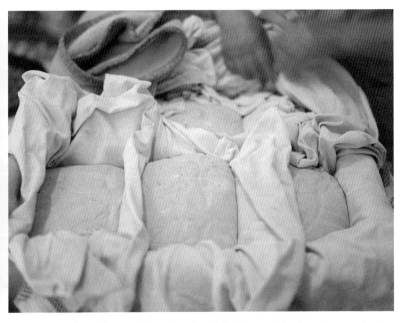

The wheat is used to make *pane al forno a legna*, bread baked in a wood-fired oven (see page 229).

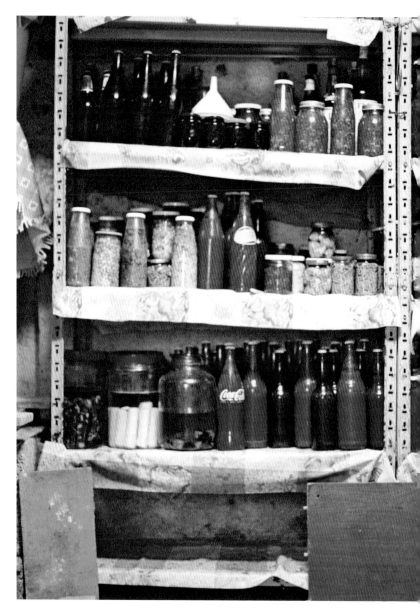

A typical Campomelano *cantina* — packed with a year's supply of home-conserved tomato sauce.

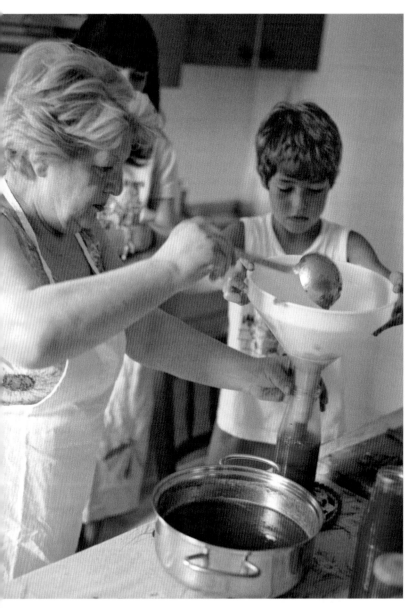

Theodora makes conserved tomato sauce with the help of her grandchildren, Martina and Lorenzo (see page 263).

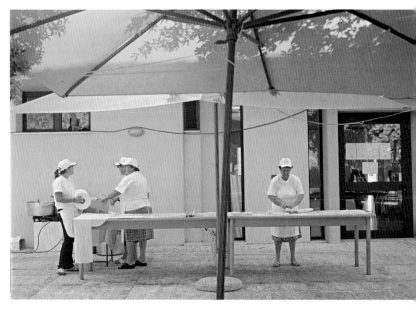

Women preparing Campodimele's traditional flour and water pasta ribbons at the annual *Laine e Fagioli* festival in August.

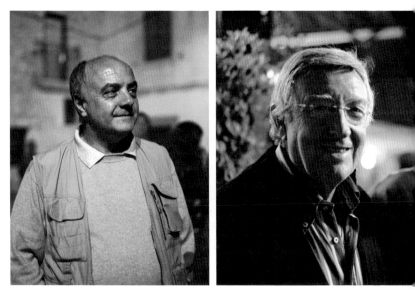

Paulo Zannella (left) and Generale Aldo Lisetti (right), former mayors of *Il Paese della Longevità*.

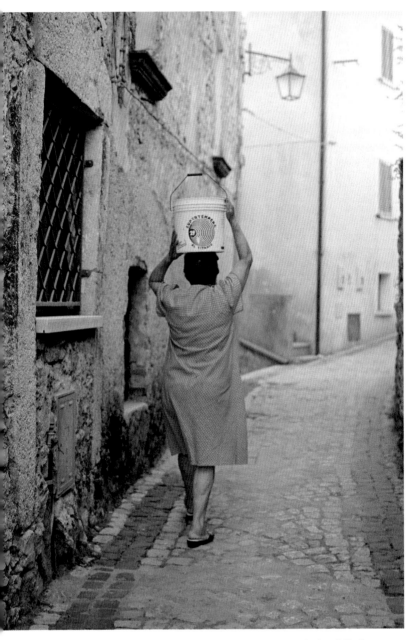

rma walks through the medieval streets of Campodimele daily, carrying water for her chilli plants.

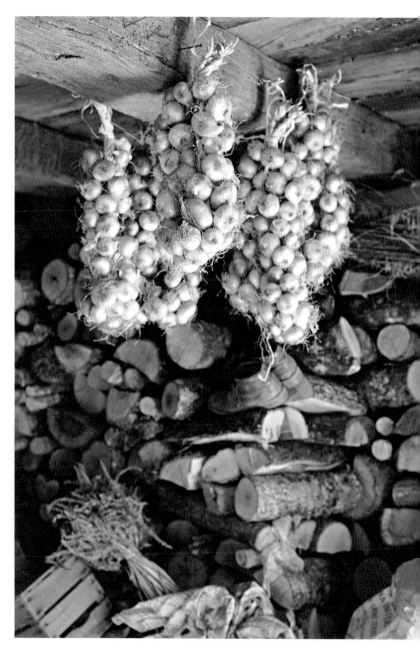

A *magazzino* stacked with logs to fuel the *forni a legna*, the wood-fired ovens in which bread and pizza are baked.

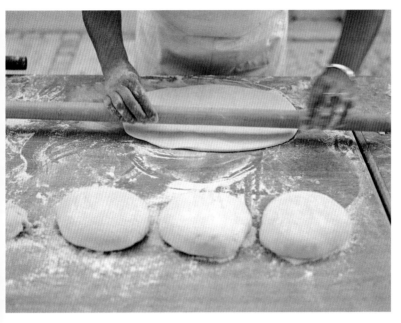

Luisa rolling out the hand-kneaded bread dough with which she makes her pizzas.

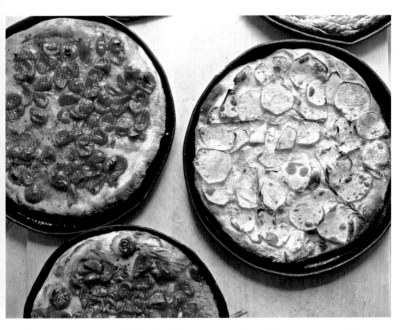

Luisa's tomato pizza (see page 318) and potato, rosemary and red chilli pizza (see pages 319).

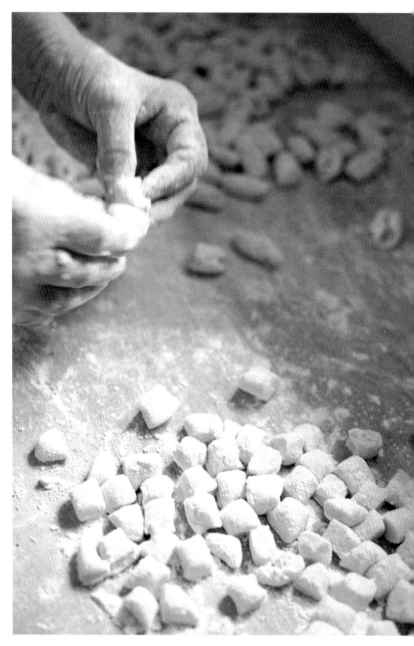

Marietta hand-crafting her potato gnocchi (see page 310).

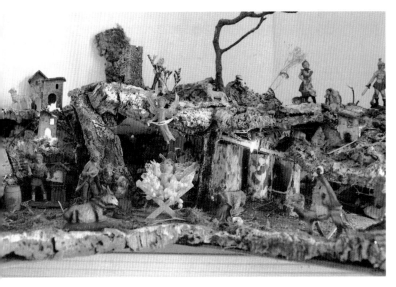

Il presepio – Gigino and Theodora's Christmas crib, the centrepiece of Italian homes in the festive season.

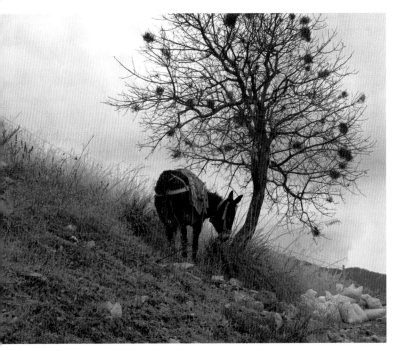

Michele and Maria's donkey waiting to transport the olive harvest, which often begins in December and continues into January.

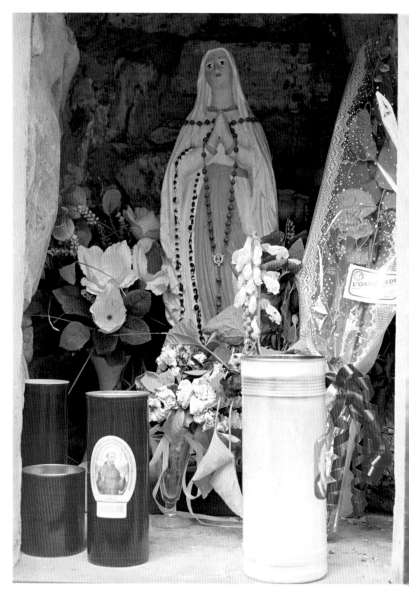

La Virgine – the shrine to the Virgin Mary on the main road into the heart of Campodimele.

Panzanella — Stale bread salad

The recipes invented to make use of days-old bread in lean times are as delicious today as they were generations ago.

Half a small loaf of slightly stale pane al forno or other coarse-
    textured bread
One small onion, thinly sliced into half-moons
Four fresh plum tomatoes, sliced lengthways into four to six segments
Four cloves of peeled garlic, squashed by the side of a knife
Handful of fresh basil leaves, torn
Few splashes of extra-virgin olive oil
Few splashes of white-wine vinegar
Fine sea salt

Rip the bread into small pieces, and place it in a large bowl along with the onion, tomatoes, garlic and basil. Mix well.

Add a few splashes of olive oil — enough to coat all the ingredients, plus a little extra, to soak into the bread.

Splash over a little white-wine vinegar, to taste. Mix well and set aside, in a cool place, for at least two hours, stirring well every now and then, to ensure the flavours meld and the bread is well moistened by the oil.

Before serving, add a little salt, to taste, and mix into the salad. This dish travels well, so can very easily be served al fresco.

Serves two.

The Meat of the Poor

This is the simplest dish, the plainest dish, the poorest dish. But it's a dish on which Campodimele grew strong, I think, as the flames catch beneath the cauldrons on the village street.

Another food festival tonight, *La Sagra di Laine e Fagioli*. *Laine*, the thin ribbons of pasta made from only flour and water; *fagioli*, the little white cannellini beans with which they are dressed. A poor man's pasta laced with poor man's meat: *la carne dei poveri*. Though tonight this pauper's dish is feted as food fit for a prince.

Festive lights arc over the piazza, stringing through the stars in the midnight sky. There's music and dancing, stalls manned by Senegalese vendors selling bangles and artefacts from far-off lands. An al fresco kitchen has been set up by Campodimele's Palazzo Culturale, and a posse of village women mix flour and water into smooth pasta mounds at outdoor tables; others roll it flat, then cut it into skinny *laine*. The beans are already dancing in huge vats of tomato *sugo*, and the sliced *laine* wriggle in boiling water for a minute or two before being drained and served up, splashed with the bean and tomato sauce.

Every *sagra* at Campodimele attracts throngs, but this one is more peopled than most because it falls just days after *Ferragosto*, the date in mid-August when Italians shut the office door, pack the car and head off for two weeks of *mare o montagna* – sea or mountains. Thousands of people throng this little mountain village tonight. Tourists from Sperlonga and Gaeta, down on the Tyrrhenian coast; sons and daughters of Campodimele who've escaped their homes in northern cities to rediscover the cooler, purer air of their childhood village. I can hear English spoken with Canadian, American, British accents – the voices of Italians born in Campodimele who left to find their fortunes abroad, and those of their children, come to discover their roots.

It's fascinating, I think, as I watch these visitors queuing for dinner, how fortunes change with time. More than any other dish I have discovered in Campodimele, nothing symbolizes *cucina povera* as unequivocally as does this dish of *laine e fagioli*. Tonight thousands of people have come up the mountain road to eat by choice a dish that was traditionally eaten here out of necessity. Because for so very long, there was little else to eat.

'*C'era la fame*,' says Pasqualina, emptying a bag of flour onto the worktop, hand-carving a volcano crater into its centre and filling the hollow with a cup of water. The *sagra* is past, the first cool days of autumn are here, and we're in her kitchen in the *centro storico*. 'There was hunger,' she repeats.

This is a phrase I hear often here, although today it's hard to imagine those difficult times.

'Those who had land could keep a pig, a few hens,' says Pasqualina, flicking cupped fingers of flour into the water, kneading for a moment or two, then repeating the action again and again. 'But most people didn't have meat, and many didn't have eggs. Instead they ate *fagioli* and *legumi*.'

Fagioli, beans, and *legumi*, pulses. Cannellini and borlotti beans, garbanzos and of course *cicerchie*. And while many a *contadino* may have lamented the lack of meat on the table, these beans and pulses have proved to hold a secret bonus. Lower in cholesterol than meat, they are credited with protecting the heart health of the Campomelani over generations. Little wonder people here live so long.

Pasqualina laughs when I say this, kneading the pasta firmly, steadily, just as she has for over seven decades. It's made from her own wheat, which is scythed annually by her daughter, Amalia, then washed and dried in the sun before being ground, bagful by bagful, at the mill in Pontecorvo.

Pasqualina, who is eighty-three now, taught herself to make *laine* as a child, so that it became her regular chore around the house. At that time this simple mix of flour and water was the only pasta she knew. *Pasta all'uovo* only became popular here after World War II, arriving in the form of lasagne and *tagliolini* from the richer north.

'We didn't even know what lasagne was when I was small,' Pasqualina says. 'If you had eggs you ate them fried. Or sold them, so you could buy something else.'

What about the third kind of pasta which is eaten here daily now, and which is also made from just flour and water: dried pasta, such as the kilometres of spaghetti and kilos of penne stockpiled in every Italian kitchen I know?

'*Si pagava un sacco di soldi!*' she says. You paid a sack of cash for dried pasta when she was young. 'They sold it loose, by the kilo, on market day, and weighed it out as you watched.' It wasn't until the easier days of the 1960s that packets of dried pasta became more affordable. Home-made *laine* remained a cheaper option. Though much more work.

Pasqualina has been pounding the pasta for twenty minutes, maybe more; turning it, flipping it, now forming it into a thick sausage. She slices off the end and holds it out to me so I can see how the flour *è sparita*, has disappeared. '*Vedi com'è bella!*' she says. 'See how beautiful it is!'

She rolls the pasta thin, thin, thin, just as she has been doing for more than seventy years, but only once or twice a month now that dried packet pasta is affordable. She rolls and turns, rolls and flips, until the pasta is a flat rectangle, then, putting her wooden pin aside, hand-rolls one flat edge of the pasta towards the centre, then hand-rolls the opposite end to meet it, shaping it like a snail with two tails. She slices through the pasta furls with a knife then unravels them into ribbons, one by one, scattering flour on the resulting tangle to prevent them sticking together.

The *laine* will need just minutes in the pan of water boiling on the cooker – two, maybe three. The beans are ready – dried cannellini which Pasqualina soaked overnight in cold water to rehydrate them, then boiled for an hour or so this morning. The *sugetto*, the little sauce, is ready too: an onion chopped and dropped into a pan full of *la bottiglia*, 'the bottle' – shorthand around here for bottled tomato conserve.

Pasqualina passes me a bowlful of drained *laine*, pours over a ladleful of *fagioli* and then splashes on the tomato sauce, flecked with the green summer basil it was bottled with. We twizzle forks in the bowls, winding the *laine* around the tines, and eat. The *laine* are thick, more weighty than the egg-rich tagliatelle they resemble, and sweet with the tomato sauce they have absorbed. Against the smoothness of the pasta the beans punctuate with what can only be described as a meaty bite.

There was hunger here. Eating *laine e fagioli* amid the excitement of the *sagra*, it's hard to imagine the difficult times. Now that the *orti* and *cantine* and tables are replete. But for those too young to remember the hungry days, or those born thousands of miles away, the memorial to Campodimele's emigrants erected outside the *centro storico* evokes those times. Its mosaic tiles depict the village's sons in fine robes, amid the accoutrements of education and leisure

– the life they found overseas. But it also portrays children dressed in rags, a thin man with an empty bowl in his hand. It's this last scene that depicts the time when *laine e fagioli* would have been eaten daily in many homes. The kind of *cucina povera* so many Campomelani, so many Italians, emigrated to escape. But which is now the basis of a celebration for which they come home.

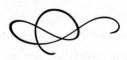

Laine e fagioli – Simple laine pasta with beans

Some people, like Pasqualina, prepare the beans and tomato sauce separately. Others set the beans to cook in the sauce, believing it helps the pulses absorb the flavour of the *odori* as they cook – I agree with them. The *guanciale* is fat from a pig's cheek and is often used to add flavour to tomato and bean sauces. Easy to come by in Italy, *guanciale* can be found at any good butcher's in the UK or the US.

For the bean sauce:
200g (7oz) dried cannellini beans or 500g (1lb 2oz) fresh
*   cannellini beans*
Pinch of bicarbonate of soda (optional)
500ml (1 pint) conserved tomato sauce (see page 263)
One golden onion, finely chopped
Strip of guanciale
Little bit of fresh basil, chopped
Handful of fresh flat-leaf parsely, chopped
Fine sea salt
Splash of extra-virgin olive oil

For the laine:
400g (14oz) '00' Doppio Zero flour
Around 200ml (7fl oz) cold water

First make the bean and tomato sauce.

If using dried beans, soak them in a large bowl of cold water for at least eight hours. Add a pinch of bicarbonate of soda to help the rehydrating process along, if desired.

Drain the beans through a colander then rinse them well under cold water.

If using fresh beans, remove them from their pods and rinse in cold water.

Bring the beans to the boil in a large pan of water, and simmer for forty minutes to an hour until al dente. The time required will depend on the size and age of the beans.

While the beans are cooking, place the tomato sauce in a pan, add the onion and the pig's cheek, and salt to taste. Simmer for fifteen minutes. (If you prefer the taste and texture of fried onions, gently fry the onion in olive oil then add the tomato sauce, pig's cheek and salt.)

Remove from the heat and add the basil and parsley.

Now make the *laine*.

Place the flour on a large, flat work surface and create a well in the centre.

Pour around 200ml (7fl oz) of water into the well then mix the pasta. To do this, curl the fingers of one hand and gently pull a little flour at a time into the water, combining each handful of flour well with the water as you go. Continue until all the flour is absorbed into the water – this may take around fifteen to twenty minutes. If the mixture becomes too dry, moisten your fingers as you go, to help it combine.

Now knead the pasta – press the heel of your palm into the end of the pasta nearest you, then pull the other end of the pasta towards you, and repeat the action. Continue this motion, turning the pasta clockwise from time to time, for around twenty minutes, until it is soft and malleable. Roll the pasta into a sausage shape and slice through the middle. If all the flour has been absorbed into the pasta, it is ready, but if you can see little pockets of flour, continue to knead until they disappear.

Wrap one half of the pasta dough in a clean, damp tea towel and set aside.

Place the other half onto a flat, lightly floured surface, and begin to roll it – turn the flattened pasta clockwise as you go, and every now and then roll it onto the rolling pin then flip it over.

When the pasta is around 3 to 4mm (⅛in) thick, lightly flour the surface and prepare to cut it into ribbons. Roll the end of the pasta sheet nearest you towards the centre then stop. Now roll the end farthest away from you towards the centre until it meets the first roll – it should resemble a snail with two tails.

Now use your sharpest knife to slice through both rolls simultaneously, to create the pasta ribbons.

Unfurl the ribbons of *laine*, ensuring they are not sticking to themselves or each other.

Unwrap the reserved half of the pasta and create a second batch of *laine* in the same way.

Now heat a large pan of boiling salted water, drop in the *laine*, and cook until they are al dente – this may take as little as two minutes, so check every twenty seconds or so to ensure they do not overcook.

While the *laine* are cooking, quickly heat the tomato and bean sauce in its pan.

Drain the cooked *laine* into a warmed bowl, and splash over a ladleful of the bean and tomato sauce. Eat immediately.

Serves four.

Fagioli conditi – Dressed beans

Many Campomelani would use only onion in this recipe, but if using the less pungent produce generally found in UK or US shops, I believe the addition of garlic adds to the flavour of these dressed beans. Because the soaking and cooking of the beans are a little time-consuming, some Campomelani cook a double or triple quantity and freeze them in small batches, adding fresh basil only when they are defrosted and reheated. The beans keep well in the freezer for at least six weeks.

200g (7oz) dried cannellini or borlotti beans
Pinch of bicarbonate of soda (optional)
Two sticks of celery
One large golden onion
Handful of fresh flat-leaf parsley
Two large cloves of garlic (optional)
Two or three splashes of extra-virgin olive oil
500ml (1 pint) conserved tomato sauce (see page 263)
Fine sea salt
Handful of fresh basil, chopped
Crushed dried red chilli (optional)

Soak the dried beans for at least eight hours in a large bowl of cold water. Add a pinch of bicarbonate of soda to help the rehydrating process along, if desired.

Finely chop the celery, onion, parsley and garlic, if using – if you have a curved-blade *mezzaluna* use that, as the more finely chopped the vegetables, the better.

Heat the olive oil in a large, deep pan, add the chopped vegetables, cover with a lid, and allow the vegetables to sweat over a low heat for around ten minutes, stirring them occasionally to ensure they do not stick to the pan.

Now drain and rinse the rehydrated beans in lots of fresh, cold water, add to the pan, and mix well with the vegetables.

Add the tomato sauce then enough water to ensure the beans are covered by around 2 to 3cm (1in).

Simmer for around forty-five minutes or more until the beans are cooked al dente and ready to eat. Add a little water now and then to ensure the beans are covered at all times, and stir frequently to ensure they don't stick to the pan.

Add salt to taste – three or four good pinches – and the fresh basil, along with the chilli, if desired. Serve hot.

Serves four to six.

Fagioli conditi con olio, aglio e prezzemolo –
Beans with oil, garlic and parsley

250g (9oz) fresh cannellini, borlotti or other beans
Pinch of bicarbonate of soda (optional)
Six cloves of garlic, peeled and squashed by the side of a knife
Four good splashes of extra-virgin olive oil
Fine sea salt
Handful of chopped fresh flat-leaf parsley (optional)

Rinse the beans thoroughly. Bring them to the boil in a pan of water. Simmer for forty-five minutes to an hour until they are al dente.

Ten minutes before the beans are ready, place the oil in a large pan, add the squashed garlic, and heat the oil, cooking the garlic gently so it chases its juices into the oil.

When the beans are ready, skim any scum from the water's surface and drain them in a colander – you can rinse a kettle of boiled water through them to eliminate any scum.

Mix the beans into the pan of garlic-infused oil, sprinkling in three or four pinches of salt, to taste.

Transfer to a serving dish and sprinkle with parsley, if using. Serve hot or cold.

Serves four to six.

Zuppa di pasta e fagioli – Pasta and bean soup

This is a wonderful, nutritious, balanced meal to come home to on a cold evening – prepare the beans in advance, and it will take just minutes to make once you have added the pasta.

One quantity of fagioli conditi made according to the recipe
*   on page 242*
400g (14oz) dried spaghetti or small pasta shapes
Handful of fresh basil, to serve
100g (3½oz) Parmigiano-Reggiano or Pecorino Romano,
*   freshly grated (optional)*

Put the *fagioli conditi* into a large, broad-based pan, and add around 250ml (½ pint) of cold water.

Heat the beans until they reach boiling point.

While waiting for the beans to boil, snap the spaghetti into 2 to 3cm (1in) pieces – or prepare the other pasta shapes.

When the beans are boiling, add the pasta to the pan, return the contents to the boil, and cook for as long as the pasta needs to become al dente, according to the instructions on the packet. Ensure there is enough liquid in the pan to cover the beans, but do not add so much that the *zuppa* becomes sloppy.

When the pasta is al dente, remove the *zuppa* from the heat and serve immediately in soup bowls.

Sprinkle with fresh basil and freshly grated Parmesan cheese or *Pecorino Romano*, if desired.

Serves four.

September

Something Hot . . .

I spotted Irma on the streets of Campodimele many times before I managed to catch her and ask her the question that was puzzling me.

Often I would round a curve on one of the lanes encircling the *centro storico* to find her walking ahead of me – then disappearing. Sometimes I'd sprint after her across a cobbled piazza, only to lose her as she slipped into a stone-stepped alleyway and out of sight. I don't imagine Irma had any idea that I was pursuing her as she strode through the village streets, or that I was eager to see her face – as opposed to her ramrod back – for the first time and ask her why she was forever balancing a big bucket on her head.

The answer, I soon discovered, was in fact all around me, at every dinner I was enjoying in every home I was invited to in Campodimele: *peperoncino*.

Peperoncino – hot chilli pepper – has been described as the 'King of *Cucina Povera*', but might better be christened the 'King of the Campodimele Kitchen', such is the reverence with which it is regarded here. *Peperoncino* is everywhere, in every season: in summer long, thin red chillies are picked fresh, chopped and fried to add a kick to pasta sauces; as autumn arrives, rotund red and green chillies are stuffed and preserved in oil; in winter and spring, strings of dried chillies hang in every home, both as amulets to attract good luck and as instant condiments to provide a blaze of heat or gentle warmth to any soup or dish. The Campomelani scatter *peperoncino* over their food as abundantly as English cooks today – and most Italian restaurants in the UK – grind black pepper over everything. It's *essenziale*, insists Peppe, the legal advisor to Campodimele's council, who is famous for carrying fresh red chillies in his shirt pocket at all times.

Peppe taught me the essential nature of *peperoncino* the hard way, when he was a guest at my first dinner party in Campodimele. Having dished up my favourite English beef and beer stew, I was puzzled when Peppe put down his fork and asked me if the string of dried chillies hanging over my fireplace was edible. When I responded yes, they were, he snapped off a chilli, whipped out a pocketknife and sliced the entire thing unapologetically over his plate. I'm not sure which of us was more astonished – me, that the beautifully mannered Peppe could do such a thing, or Peppe, that I could serve up a meal without a scrap of *peperoncino* in the mix.

While black pepper is universally associated with Italian cuisine, it is not native to Italy – it came to the peninsula from the East. It may have seduced the Roman Empire and the northern regions with its tangy warmth, but its relatively high price tag – indeed the fact it had to be paid for at all – meant it never gained a foothold in Campodimele. In leaner times money could be better spent on other things. Today few feel inclined to add what are generally regarded as lukewarm black pepper grains to their store-cupboard when they can grow something more fiery and versatile in their own vegetable gardens. Besides, *pepe nero fa male*, everyone here exclaims – black pepper is bad for you – and I've failed to convince anyone that scientists are finding evidence to the contrary. Though I am happy to accept the philosophy that *peperoncino fa bene* – *peperoncino* is good for you – especially for the immune system.

This is the explanation for Irma's daily pilgrimage through the village balancing a big bucket on her head: water for chillies. From her home on Via Roma she negotiates cobbled lanes and stone staircases, balancing around 20 litres of water atop her rich red curls. '*Non è pesante*' – 'It's not heavy' – she assures me when I finally catch up with her, and before I know it she is grabbing my carrier bag of shopping with her right hand, balancing the bucket with the fingers of her left and flashing me a smile that tells me to take it easy.

Irma cultivates her chilli peppers at *le galline*, the hen houses which sprawl to the east of the village. As she splashes water onto the roots of her plants, she tells me she's been raising chillies here since she was married at the age of twenty-six and moved to Campodimele from the outlying countryside. Her plants are lush bushes of tropical green leaves which overflow from old oil canisters and outsized aluminium pans. Irma grows three kinds of chillies: a tiny but fiery red variety; their longer, thinner, milder red cousins; and the *peperoncino rotondo* – rotund chillies whose deep bellies are perfect for Irma's speciality, *peperoncini ripieni*: stuffed chillies.

The chillies dangle like gemstones, dazzlingly red and green, and look ripe for the plucking. But not today. '*Aspetto la luna calante*' – 'I'm waiting for the waning moon' – she explains in a tone that conveys I'm mad to even suggest picking chillies when the moon is still waxing. '*Non vengono buoni!*' she warns me. 'They won't come good!'

Like Irma, many villagers still adhere to the ancient practice of sowing and reaping according to the phases of the moon. But I've found one crazy person prepared to supply me with a few of the rotund fireballs, and Irma, whose stuffed chillies are famous in these parts, has agreed to show me what to do with them. Although the expression on her face suggests she doesn't hold out much hope for the savouriness of these untimely specimens.

In the cool of her kitchen, where women have been preparing food for hundreds of years, Irma lays out the ingredients with which she will stuff her *peperoncini ripieni*: capers, tuna, anchovies, olives. She snaps on thin rubber gloves to keep the fire of the chillies from her skin and slices off their lids with a knife, tipping out the seeds. She sprinkles the insides of the chillies with finely ground sea salt and white vinegar. Then she spoons a few capers into each of the chilli bellies, stuffing flakes of tinned tuna on top. Next she wraps an anchovy fillet around a stoned green olive and squashes it into the neck of the chilli to plug it. The chillies will be slotted into jars which will be filled with olive oil and stored in her *cantina* down the street, a storehouse whose shelves are lined with tomato sauce, sausage in oil, garlands of onions, piles of potatoes. In a few months the flavours of the stuffing will meld with the fiery flesh encasing them. The peppers will serve as instant antipasti or maybe even as a *contorno*, mouthfuls of inert heat which once bitten will explode with complex layers of fiery flavours in the mouth.

Or will they? Having been picked out of time, in the wrong phase of the moon, will they really fail to come good?

Irma smiles, screwing a lid onto the glass jar in which the chillies will be preserved. 'Let's leave them a while,' she says. 'Then you'll see what I mean.'

But why does the phase of the moon make such a difference? And how?

Irma shrugs.

'*Così*,' she responds, '*sempre così.*' That's the way it is, the way it's always been. And sometimes, that's reason enough. A reverence for tradition, faith in the mystery of Nature's gifts. The understanding that sometimes we have no answers. That questions need not be asked.

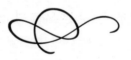

Peperoncini sott'olio – Peperoncini preserved in oil

This is a useful way of preserving chillies to ensure you always have a ready supply to add to dishes.

Twelve red or green fresh chillies
Roughly 100ml (3fl oz) white-wine vinegar
Roughly 150ml (5fl oz) extra-virgin olive oil
500ml (1 pint) glass jar with screw top, sterilized (see page 188)

Wearing rubber gloves, wash and dry the chillies then finely slice them and place in a shallow bowl.

Splash with enough white-wine vinegar to ensure all the chillies are coated, and leave to soak in the vinegar for about forty-eight hours, stirring regularly.

After forty-eight hours, drain the chillies in a colander and rinse with cold water. Dry thoroughly using a clean tea towel or kitchen paper then spread out in a cool, dry environment and allow to dry further for an hour or two.

Pour a little olive oil into the bottom of the jar, add the chillies to within 1cm (½in) of the top of the jar, and fill with olive oil, tilting the jar to ensure no air pockets remain. Ensure the chillies are covered with oil before sealing, and store in a cool, dark place. Once opened, they should be stored in the fridge and used within two months. As you use them, ensure the chillies are not exposed to air by topping up with olive oil as you go.

Makes about one 500ml (1 pint) jar of chillies.

Peperoncini ripieni – Stuffed chilli peppers

You will need two or three glass storage jars with airtight lids to preserve these chillies, and these must be sterilized by washing in very hot soapy water then dried in the oven at a low heat (see page 188). The size of your chillies will dictate the number of jars you fill.

Twenty small round-bellied chillies – red or green, according to taste
Fine sea salt
200ml (7fl oz) white-wine vinegar
200g (7oz) jar of capers in white-wine vinegar
400g (14oz) jar of tuna fillets preserved in olive oil
Twenty anchovy fillets
Twenty green olives, stones removed
Around three 300ml (10fl oz) glass jars with screw tops, sterilized
Around 1 litre (2 pints) extra-virgin olive oil, depending on the
   sizes of the chillies

Wash and dry the chillies then slice off their tops and remove and discard the white seeds and pith inside.

Sprinkle fine sea salt and vinegar into the belly of each chilli then place them in a bowl in a cool place overnight, to allow the salt to remove the bitter juices.

The next day, rinse out the salt and stand the chillies upside down on a dry tablecloth to allow them to dry.

When the insides are dry, spoon a few capers into the bottom of each chilli, followed by a spoonful of tuna fillet. Then wrap an anchovy fillet around one of the stoned olives and slip it into the neck of the chilli to plug it. Place the chilli in the bottom of one of the sterilized glass jars. Continue doing this until the jar is nearly full – leave a 1cm (½in) gap between the top of the uppermost chillies and the neck of the jar.

Next pour olive oil into the jar, tilting the jar to work the oil into all the cracks and to eliminate air bubbles. The chillies must be totally covered with oil.

Seal the jar and leave in a cool, dark place for a few weeks to allow the flavours to meld.

After opening a jar to eat some of the chillies, top up with olive oil ensuring the remaining ones are completely covered with oil, to preserve them. Once opened, the jar should be kept in the fridge and the chillies should be consumed quickly.

Makes about three 300ml (10fl oz) jars of chillies.

Spaghetti con olio, aglio e peperoncino –
Spaghetti with garlic, olive oil and hot chilli pepper

This spaghetti dish is known in Campodimele as the spaghetti of cuckolds because it's so quick to make that it's the pasta course of choice for housewives too busy being unfaithful to their husbands to prepare anything more elaborate. It is indeed the simplest and most delicious store-cupboard standby meal.

400g (14oz) spaghetti
Three or four good splashes of extra-virgin olive oil
Three cloves of the freshest garlic, finely chopped
Fine sea salt
Few good pinches of crushed dried red chilli

Bring a large pan of salted water to the boil, add the spaghetti, and cook according to the instructions on the packet – usually about eight to ten minutes.

About one minute before the pasta is cooked al dente, heat the olive oil in a large, deep pan and add the garlic – stir over a high heat for about one minute, ensuring the garlic does not colour.

Remove the oil and garlic from the heat, and stir in a pinch or two of salt and a few pinches of crushed dried chilli – add a little or a lot, according to taste.

The spaghetti should now be al dente, so drain through a colander, and add to the pan of flavoured oil, mixing well to ensure every strand is well coated.

Serves four.

Penne all'arrabbiata –
Penne pasta with chilli-tomato sauce

Arrabbiato is the Italian word for 'angry' – how angry depends on how much chilli you add to this dish.

400g (14oz) dried penne pasta
Good splash of extra-virgin olive oil
Two cloves of garlic, finely chopped
Half a small, fresh red chilli or a good sprinkling of crushed dried
    red chilli
500ml (1 pint) conserved tomato sauce (see page 263)
Fine sea salt
Handful of fresh flat-leaf parsley, finely chopped
100g (3½oz) freshly grated Parmigiano-Reggiano or Pecorino
    Romano (optional)

Bring a large pan of salted water to the boil, add the penne, and cook according to the instructions on the packet.

About four minutes before the penne are al dente, heat the olive oil in a large, deep pan then add the garlic and fresh chilli, if using, and stir for about a minute – take care that the garlic does not burn. If using dried chilli, add to the pan once the garlic has cooked for a minute.

Add the tomato sauce and a good pinch of sea salt, to taste. Bring gently to the boil, and lower the heat to a gentle simmer.

When the penne are cooked al dente, drain them and stir them into the pan containing the sauce. Serve immediately, with the chopped parsley and the grated cheese, if desired.

Serves four.

The Bottle

The clashing of glass has been everywhere these past few days. It rattles in old tin oil drums suspended over gas stoves on cobbled streets; it clinks in aluminium vats which bubble on kitchen cookers; it tinkles in plastic carrier bags lugged through the village and emptied into stone-shelved *cantine*.

The tomato glut is here and with it the annual ritual which, perhaps more than any other, encapsulates the Campomelano practice of fast food, slow style: *la conservazione dei pomodori* – the conserving of tomato sauce.

The scale of the activity is immense: mountains of tomatoes are being brought in from the fields; oceans of red sauce are being set to bubble in outsized pans; hundreds of glass jars are being squashed into a single kitchen. It seems that everybody in every corner of the village is harvesting, cooking and bottling tomatoes, scenting the air with their sun-sugared sweetness.

'*Quattro quintali*,' smiles Leana outside her stone-walled house with its geranium-strewn staircase. Four hundred kilos, around four thousand tomatoes to clean, chop and boil.

Leana got up at 3.30 a.m. yesterday to begin *la conservazione* and has worked for sixteen hours a day over two days to complete the process and stock her larder with around 350 bottles of *sugo*. Her weekend has been a logistical marathon, but the tomatoes are in their prime, sweet beyond measure after months of sun, and if they are not harvested and conserved right now, they will spoil on the vine.

My friend Theodora takes a more relaxed, but equally systematic, approach, devoting five mornings of a single week to preserving tomatoes which are bought, but – and this is crucial – *della zona*, from the area around Campodimele, so fresh off the plant and unlikely to be laced with chemicals. Today she has enlisted the help of her son, Francesco, twenty-four, and her grandchildren Martina, thirteen, and Lorenzo, nine, not just because this is hard work, but because she is keen that her family maintain this tradition.

'*Cibo genuino, niente conservanti*,' shrugs Theodora. 'Genuine food, no preservatives', save for a little salt and the natural preserving power of the heating process. Considering the amount of tomato sauce Italians consume, it's easy to understand why any grandmother is happiest to see her family consuming the home-made stuff.

Martina is keen to learn too. 'I've eaten factory-made tomato sauce at friends' houses before and it just doesn't taste this good,' she says, lining up sterilized glass jars on the kitchen table and dropping a basil leaf into each one, to lend a summery perfume to the sauce.

Theodora is making two different kinds of preserved tomato sauce: *cotto*, cooked, and *crudo*, raw. She's chosen San Marzano, the classic tomato used in Italian sauces, and Roma, another popular choice. At their ripest, these tomatoes are also delicious chopped raw with basil and garlic as a coating for spaghetti on a hot day.

But not today.

'Discard any which have broken skins because they can be acidic,' Theodora advises, picking through the pile of tomatoes. 'And there might be insects inside.' Scooping out the eyes of the tomatoes with a knife, she slices the fruit in half and piles them into a huge aluminium pan with nothing other than a good sprinkling of salt. She boils them over a high heat for an hour and a quarter, until much of the water has evaporated from the tomatoes, resulting in a thick *sugo*. Then Lorenzo balances a funnel over each jar as his grandmother ladles in rivers of boiling-hot red sauce, filling each one almost to the top then sealing it with a screw-top lid. Theodora places the jars in plastic crates which are lined in newspaper and woollen blankets, where they will take almost a day to cool.

Meanwhile Martina and Lorenzo have devised their production line for the *sugo crudo*. Martina slices two raw tomatoes lengthways into quarters, drops them into a jar then hands it to her brother. Lorenzo mashes the raw fruit with the handle of a wooden spoon, hands the jar back to Martina, and the process begins again. Lorenzo sighs as the jar fills up and the mashing process becomes harder and harder. Will he continue this tradition when he is grown up, as *Nonna* Theodora hopes? '*Se mi pagano!*' he responds. 'If they pay me!'

Unlike those bottled straight from the bubbling pan, these tomatoes are raw and so must be sterilized in their sealed jars to eliminate the possibility of botulism. This vital step is achieved through heat processing with the aid of a *bagnomaria*, what the French and anglophones call a *bain-marie*. Theodora arranges the jars in a large aluminium pan and covers them with cold water. She brings the water to a boil, leaving it to bubble for at least forty-five minutes, so rendering the cooked tomatoes hygienic and safe to eat for a year.

This raw sauce retains the water and much of the structure of the tomatoes, and will be used in dishes which require lengthy cooking or texture, such as *fave in umido*, stewed broad beans, or as an oven-baked pizza topping. The thicker cooked sauce sheds most of its water during cooking so is ideal for adding concentrated flavour to meat *ragù* in the last fifteen minutes of cooking, or as a sauce for pasta.

Some cooks squeeze the sauce through a food mill before bottling it, to eliminate the skin and seeds, resulting in *passata*, which literally means 'passed'. Theodora usually does this *al momento* – just when the bottles of sauce are opened and about to be used. Today, though, she boils up a second pan of tomatoes, splashes the hot sauce into a metal *mulino per verdure*, turning the handle so that the *sugo* emerges like liquid velvet, ready to be bottled and sterilized in the *bagnomaria* because it has cooled in the milling process.

The conserved sauce looks fabulous: cratefuls of summer ripeness in Theodora's kitchen, shelves full of tomato red flecked with basil green in Leana's *cantina*. But this has been time-consuming: two days out of Leana's life, five mornings out of Theodora's week. Wouldn't it be quicker to cook up a fresh tomato sauce as and when required, even if the winter fruits have been grown under artificial light and lack the sweetness of the summer crop?

No, says Theodora, who would not dream of a summer passing by without this ritual conserving of sauce. Aside from the all-important fact that this is healthy and delicious *cibo genuino*, it has given her a larder full of instant tomato sauce – the Campodimele equivalent of the so-called fresh pasta sauces for sale in supermarkets, but minus the additives and at a fraction of the cost. It encapsulates perfectly the convenient aspect of the Campodimele kitchen: devote a day or two to preserving now, and you can enjoy the benefits of your labour all year round.

At nine years old, Lorenzo struggles to appreciate the value of this.

'*Nonna, dove trovi questa forza?*' he cries as he endeavours to mash two more raw tomatoes into their glass jar. 'Where do you find the strength?'

Theodora smiles. It is the smile of a million Italian *nonne*, for whom no kitchen task is too tiresome or too time-consuming if it benefits her family's palate or health.

'*Dove trovo l'amore, trovo la forza!*' she replies. 'Where I find love, I find strength!'

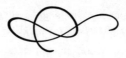

Sugo cotto in bottiglia — Cooked conserved tomato sauce

1 o kilos of tomatoes makes about 1 o litres of cooked sauce, though the amount you realize will depend both on the water content of the tomatoes and on how much water evaporates before they are bottled. The salt is an aid to preserving the tomatoes, so don't skimp. This recipe removes much of the water from the sauce, so is ideal for adding to meat *ragù* in the last fifteen minutes of cooking or for use as an instant pasta sauce.

10kg (22lb) freshest, ripest organic tomatoes
Ten good pinches of fine sea salt
Ten 1 litre (2 pint) glass jars with screw tops
Ten large, fresh basil leaves, thoroughly washed

Thoroughly wash the tomatoes.

Discard any tomatoes which have breaks in the skin – these can be acidic and might harbour insects.

Roughly chop the tomatoes then place them in a pan and gradually bring to a rapid boil.

Add a good pinch of salt for every kilo or couple of pounds of tomatoes – this will help the preserving process as well as the taste.

Lower the heat slightly, but keep the tomatoes bubbling and cook for a further hour and fifteen minutes, until much of the water has evaporated, resulting in a thick, red sauce.

While the sauce is cooking, sterilize the glass jars and funnel according to the instructions on page 188.

Place a basil leaf in the bottom of each of the jars.

When the sauce is thick and making slurping sounds, place the sterilized funnel over a jar and ladle the boiling-hot sauce directly into it. Close the lid tightly the moment the jar has filled, to prevent bacteria entering the bottle.

If the temperature of the sauce drops before you have time to bottle it, take the extra hygiene precaution of heating the sealed bottles in a *bagnomaria* to limit the risk of food poisoning (see page 266).

Place the glass jars in a crate or cardboard box lined with newspapers and an old woollen blanket which overlaps the sides – then place a few layers of newspaper on top and pull the overlapping blanket across the top of the crate, covering the jars. Retaining the heat in this way is considered a vital part of the sterilizing process in Campodimele. The bottles will still be warm twenty-four hours later.

Once the bottles have fully cooled, store them in a cool, dark place. Reach for *la bottiglia* whenever you need to! If furring occurs in any of the jars, throw them and their contents out.

Makes around 10 litres (20 pints) of sauce.

Sugo di pomodori crudi in bottiglia –
Raw conserved tomato sauce

As with the previous recipe for cooked conserved tomato
sauce, thoroughly sterilized jars are essential. The raw
conserve retains the water content and more of the texture
of the tomatoes, so is more suitable when cooking at high
temperatures, such as when baking pizza, or when you are
looking for more texture in a *ragù* or pasta sauce – in which
case you will need to allow time for the water to evaporate
a little in the finished dish.

20kg (22lb) freshest, ripest organic tomatoes – preferably San
   Marzano or Roma
Thirty 500ml (1 pint) glass jars with screw tops
Thirty large basil leaves, thoroughly washed

Thoroughly wash the tomatoes.

Thoroughly sterilize the glass jars and a wooden spoon
(see page 188).

Place a basil leaf in each of the jars. Now slice two
tomatoes lengthways into halves or quarters, and place
them into a jar. Mash the tomatoes with the handle end of
the wooden spoon, to create more space in the jar. Then
slice another two tomatoes into halves or quarters, put
them in the jar and mash. Repeat this process until the jar is
almost full. Immediately screw-top.

When all the jars are full, stand them upright in a large
pan as the first step of the *bagnomaria* process – you may
have to do this in two or three batches.

Fill the pan with enough cold water to completely cover the jars. Bring the water to the boil, and boil the jars for around sixty minutes.

When the jars have boiled for at least an hour, carefully tip the boiling water from the pan, and remove the jars. Dry them and place them in a crate or box lined with newspapers and, if possible, a woollen blanket. Wrap them well and leave to cool over the next day or so.

When the tomatoes have cooled, store them in a cool, dark place and enjoy whenever the mood takes you.

Makes roughly 15 litres (30 pints) of sauce.

Spaghetti ai pomodori freschi e crudi —
Spaghetti with fresh raw tomato sauce

This cold sauce using raw tomatoes is the perfect antidote to a searing summer's day. Much of the sauce is made up of olive oil, so be sure to use your finest.

500g (1lb) ripest, fresh organic plum tomatoes —
*   San Marzano or Roma are the best*
Few good splashes of best extra-virgin olive oil
Handful of fresh basil, torn
Handful of fresh parsley, finely chopped
One clove of garlic, very finely chopped
Finely ground sea salt
400g (14oz) spaghetti

Skin and deseed the tomatoes, and chop the flesh finely.

Place the chopped tomatoes in a bowl along with a few good splashes of olive oil, the herbs and garlic. Marinate at room temperature for at least fifteen minutes.

Set a large pan of salted water to boil. When it is bubbling, add the spaghetti. Return to the boil again, and cook according to the instructions on the packet – usually eight to ten minutes.

When the spaghetti is cooked al dente, drain into a colander then return to the cooking pan, add the sauce, and stir gently with two forks to ensure every strand is coated. Add salt to taste. Serve immediately.

Serves four.

Penne al sugo fresco di pomodori –
Pasta with fresh tomato sauce

This warm tomato sauce takes just fifteen minutes to make and is an everyday alternative to conserving your own tomatoes: many people here make it in summer ahead of *la conservazione* if their supply of bottled tomatoes is running low and fresh tomatoes are already ripe on the plant. If your tomatoes are not ripe as ripe can be (often the case with imports), add a pinch of sugar to counter any acidity.

1kg (2lb 3oz) ripest, fresh organic tomatoes – Piccadilly is often the variety of choice for this sauce in Campodimele
Good splash of extra-virgin olive oil
Two or three large cloves of garlic, peeled and crushed by the side of a knife
400g (14oz) penne or other pasta
Fine sea salt
Four large basil leaves, torn, and a few smaller leaves, to garnish
100g (3½oz) finely grated Parmigiano-Reggiano or Pecorino Romano (optional)

Roughly chop the tomatoes.

Splash some extra-virgin olive oil into a broad-based, deep pan and add the garlic. Heat gently until the garlic begins to sizzle, but do not let it colour – you just want the oil to take on its flavour.

Add the tomatoes to the pan, bring to the boil then reduce to a rapid simmer for about ten minutes, so the water from the tomatoes evaporates to leave a thick sauce.

When the pasta sauce is thick and almost ready, start to cook the pasta – bring a large pan of salted water to the boil, add the pasta, and cook according to the instructions on the packet – usually around eight to ten minutes.

When the tomato sauce is so thick that it is making slurping sounds, throw in the torn large basil leaves – reserving the smaller ones for garnish – and salt to taste. Simmer on a low heat until the pasta is al dente.

When the pasta is ready, drain it in a colander and throw into the pan of sauce, mixing gently with two forks to ensure all the pasta is coated.

Serve immediately in warmed bowls, sprinkled with the cheese and a fresh basil leaf or two, if desired.

Serves four.

Summer Suspended

Until a few decades ago here, fresh ingredients for lunch meant gathering whatever was ripe in your *orto* that day, or what you could forage on the mountainside. But modern agriculture and transport links mean that even in Campodimele, a village whose heart beats to the rhythms of Nature, seasonal boundaries can sometimes be blurred.

I realized this when I arrived here in the depths of winter. January mists hid the mountainside and the valley floor, rendering Campodimele a kingdom in the air. Wind screeched like an angry serpent along ancient alleys and rain spat from a sunless sky. The soil of the *orti* was saturated black, punctuated by the dark shadows of *broccoletti* and *cavolo nero*, the staple winter greens. Amid this subdued landscape there was one oasis of colour outdoors – the *frutta verdura*.

Frutta verdura means 'fruit and vegetables', and is the Italian name for shops which sell fresh produce. Campodimele does not have a *frutta verdura* of its own, but on Wednesdays and Fridays Franco and Anna drive their fruit-and-vegetable wagon up from Fondi to sell their produce, valued here because much of it is *della zona*, 'from the zone'.

On those first grey January days the *frutta verdura* sometimes seemed the only source of brightness in the village, with its piles of red tomatoes and ranks of golden melons. Right away I noticed that many people were happily taking these out-of-season splashes of sunshine home. However, others – especially the older residents – were filling their shopping baskets only with winter produce. Or, put another way, seasonal produce.

Assunta is typical of the latter. She goes to the *frutta verdura* for food which she can't get home-grown here, and produce which doesn't grow in Campodimele – lemons from Sicily and the fabulous oranges from Fondi – winter fruits which don't thrive in these cooler mountain climes.

'*Ma sempre in stagione!*' she insists. 'Always in season!' To Assunta seasonal cooking is instinctive, a way of life she grew up with and which she would never question. As she expresses it, seasonal eating just makes sense.

Now it's September, it's the season for eating peppers, and because she doesn't grow them Assunta is buying them by the basketful from the *frutta verdura*. The capsicums are huge, twice the size of her palm, their irregular forms writhing with vigour, their shiny red and yellow skins streaked with green.

'*In padella con aglio e prezzemolo . . . in padella con melanzane . . . nel forno, poi condito con olio, aglio e prezzemolo . . .*' Assunta lists the ways she serves fresh peppers in season: in the pan with garlic and parsley . . . in the pan with aubergines . . . oven-roasted then dressed with olive oil, garlic and parsley . . . '*Ti faccio assaggiare!*' she promises. 'I'll make some for you to taste!' Campomelani are never happier than when feeding people.

But the pile of peppers in Assunta's kitchen is not for eating today; it's for preserving and consuming later – the one form of unseasonal eating which is universally acceptable here. Assunta has dragged a demijohn into her kitchen, a huge glass jar with a bowled body and narrow neck, with an outer coating of plastic mesh to protect it from bumps and knocks. The room reeks of red-wine vinegar, which she has mixed with water and poured into the demi-john. She washes the peppers and slips them one by one into the jar, placing them carefully so as to squeeze in as many as possible. A lid on the jar and that's the peppers preserved, ready to be sliced and eaten with salads or as a side dish next month or next year – whenever they are required.

It seems astonishingly quick and easy, peppers which are stall-bought but home-processed, a marriage of the commercial and the *casereccio*, a countryside tradition I can imagine recreating effortlessly in an urban setting. But I can't help wondering why these peppers, having been purchased, not produced on Assunta's land, are worth preserving at all. Why not just trot down to the *frutta verdura* in the winter and buy them when she wants them for lunch?

'*Perché d'inverno non sono in stagione!*' – 'Because in winter they are not in season!' Seasonality, she adds, being the key.

This is for many reasons: food bought in season is likely to be *della zona*, and so fresh as fresh can be, not imported from the warmer south or – even worse – from outside Italy. This means it is less likely to be saturated with preservatives. And you'll pay a sack of cash for them in the winter, she adds, with the unabashed thriftiness of the Italian housewife who knows that if you buy fruit and vegetables when they are in glut, they cost a fraction of what they do even a week or two later. But, even more importantly, there is the question of taste. '*Sono ottime adesso,*' says Assunta. 'They're at their best just now,' she says, 'The ones you buy in the winter never taste this good.'

'*Ogni cosa ha il suo momento*' – 'Everything has its time,' concludes Assunta, quoting the mantra of the *contadino*, the philosophy of those who work with and respect the land. And just as the best moment for in-season food is now, when it's fresh off the plant, so the best moment for out-of-season food is also now – picking the produce at its flavoursome peak then preserving it in vinegar or oil, suspending a little piece of summer in time to savour amid the winter chill: making non-seasonal eating seasonal after all.

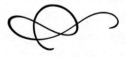

Peperonata — Stewed sweet peppers

Three good splashes of extra-virgin olive oil
Two cloves of garlic, peeled and crushed by the side of a knife
One large red pepper, deseeded and sliced
One large yellow pepper, deseeded and sliced
One small golden onion, sliced into fine rounds
Fine sea salt
Handful of flat-leaf parsley, finely chopped
Handful of fresh basil leaves
Crushed dried red chilli (optional)

Place the oil in a deep frying pan along with the garlic, and heat the oil gently, allowing the garlic to impart its flavour into it. Do not let the garlic colour and burn.

Add the peppers and onions along with a good pinch of sea salt, and fry gently for around twenty to thirty minutes, stirring frequently to make sure the peppers do not burn. If the garlic starts to burn, remove it from the pan and discard.

When the peppers and onions are soft and melting, sprinkle over the parsley and basil, stir well then add a few pinches of chilli, if using. Taste for salt, and add more if desired.

Serve hot, with lots of fresh crusty bread – although this dish tastes more delicious the following day, served at room temperature.

Serves four as a side dish.

Insalata di peperoni arrostiti – Roasted sweet-pepper salad

Four red peppers – yellow peppers work well too
Handful of fresh flat-leaf parsley, finely chopped
Handful of fresh basil, torn into small pieces
Two cloves of garlic, very finely sliced
Fine sea salt
Four good splashes of extra-virgin olive oil

Preheat the oven to around 200°C/400°F/Gas Mark 6 then place the peppers in a shallow baking dish and roast for around twenty-five to thirty minutes, or until their skins are black. Alternatively, grill the peppers over an open flame.

Remove from the oven and, while still hot, peel away the skins – if you place the roasted peppers in a sealed polythene bag for around fifteen minutes, it will be easier to remove the skins.

Slice the peeled peppers and place on a serving plate.

Sprinkle over the parsley, basil and finely sliced garlic, sprinkle with salt to taste, and drizzle with plenty of olive oil.

This salad is at its best if left for at least an hour or so at room temperature, to allow the flavours to meld.

Serves four.

Peperoni e melanzane imbottiti –
Sweet peppers and aubergines stuffed and stewed

This is a hearty main-course dish that uses stale bread to stuff the peppers – a legacy from the days of *cucina povera* when nothing was thrown away.

Four large peppers – two red and two yellow
Two aubergines – the round kind, suitable for stuffing, preferably
  ones whose juices do not need extracting due to bitterness
Three large, thick-cut slices of stale bread, shredded
Three fresh organic eggs, lightly beaten
150g (5oz) Parmigiano-Reggiano or Pecorino Romano, freshly
  grated
Handful of green olives, stoned and chopped
Few pinches of fine sea salt
Around twelve plum tomatoes, skinned, deseeded and chopped
Large handful of fresh basil leaves, torn
Four cloves of garlic, peeled and squashed by the side of a knife
Six or seven good splashes of extra-virgin olive oil
750ml (1 ½ pints) conserved tomato sauce (see page 263)

Slice the stalks then the tops off the peppers, remove the seeds and sprinkle a little salt around the insides of the shells.

Remove the green leaves from the aubergines and slice off the tops. Using a sharp knife, slice into the interior of the aubergines to scoop out the innards, being sure not to pierce the skin. Continue until they are hollowed out.

In a bowl, mix the aubergine innards, shredded stale bread, eggs, Parmesan, olives, salt, tomatoes and half the basil. Chop one of the garlic cloves finely, add and mix. Use this mixture to stuff the peppers and aubergines. Pack them well, because the bread will lose much of its volume during the stewing process.

Squash the 'lids' back onto the peppers and aubergines, fixing them in place lightly with a toothpick or two, or a metal skewer.

Pour the olive oil into a large, broad-based pan along with the remaining garlic cloves, and heat gently. When the oil is hot, lay the peppers and aubergines sideways in the pan in a single layer and cover with a lid. Cook gently over a low flame for around an hour, turning the peppers and aubergines frequently to ensure they cook evenly on all sides.

After an hour, pour the tomato conserve into the pan, mixing it well with the cooking oil. Continue to cook gently, turning the peppers and aubergines frequently for a further hour, or until the pepper shells are soft.

Serve hot or at room temperature, splashed with the cooking juices and a little extra basil.

Serves six.

Peperoni e peperoncini sott'aceto –
Sweet red peppers and chilli peppers preserved in vinegar

This recipe requires a wide-necked storage jar large enough to hold as many peppers and chillies as you wish to preserve.

Around twelve medium-sized sweet red peppers
Around twelve small red chilli peppers
Around 1 litre (2 pints) red-wine vinegar
Around 1 litre (2 pints) water which has been boiled and allowed
    to cool in a covered container
8 litre (16 pint) glass jar with screw lid, sterilized (see page 188)
Large pan, sterilized

Wash the sweet peppers and chillies thoroughly then place a layer of peppers in the bottom of the sterilized jar, followed by a layer of chillies and a layer of peppers. Continue layering until the jar is almost full – leave a gap of around 4cm (2in) between the peppers and the top of the jar.

Combine the red-wine vinegar and boiled water in the sterilized pan then, holding the peppers down in the jar with a wooden spoon, pour the liquid into the jar until it covers the peppers – fill almost to the top, ensuring all the peppers are covered. Seal tightly.

Store in a cool, dark place for at least three weeks before using the peppers, to allow them to absorb the flavour of the vinegar. These should keep well for at least six months.

Serve sliced with salads, or as antipasti, drizzled with olive oil, salt, fresh-leaf parsley and basil.

Makes one 8 litre (16 pint) jar of peppers.

OCTOBER

Under the Pergola, In the Orchard

There's a scent of strawberries here, a ruby ripeness on the autumn air. So strong that it sweeps me home to English summer teas, jugs of cream, tennis on trim green lawns. But there's not a strawberry to be seen. Only the grapes burgeoning on the vine.

'*Uva fragola*,' says Pasqualina, plucking one of the purple globes and passing it to me. It tastes like strawberry coulis laced with red wine. So this is the strawberry grape, I think, understanding its Italian name for the first time.

The vines are heavy with *uva fragola* just now. They dangle from pergolas to bask in the sweetening sun. Pasqualina has trained her vine onto a fence into which she's cut a low archway, and as you step through, the *uva fragola* brush against your skin and bruise it with their juices. She snips me a *grappolo*, a handful, of grapes. It's surprisingly heavy, but then it's straight off the plant and its juice has not had a chance to evaporate yet.

'*Uva da tavola*,' Pasqualina goes on, 'grapes for the table.' And she tells me to eat them today, while they are perfectly ripe, as *la frutta*, the fruit course of my lunch.

Frutta is the final course of an everyday lunch or dinner in Italy and as essential as the *primo*, the *secondo* with its accompanying *contorno* and the palate-cleansing third course of *insalata*.

Many fruit trees survive the cold and damp of winter here: cherries arrive towards the end of spring, then apricots with their sunset blush, and purple mulberries. As summer fades there are apples and pears and the stickiest of figs. And in the colder months there are *cachi*, the fiery orange persimmons, and *mele cotogne*, quinces.

And then in late autumn there is *frutta secca*, which translates as 'dried fruit', but which is the term used here for nuts – walnuts, which are turned into *nocciola* liqueur, and sweet almonds, smashed and eaten along with fresh fruit. Further up the mountains, I'm told, wild strawberries grow in late spring and summer, smaller and sweeter than those grown in the *orti*. But there are also wild dogs which roam in a pack, so it's wiser to leave the wild strawberries to the birds.

Like the *uva da tavola*, almost all these fruits are eaten fresh, raw, uncooked, unadulterated. Or preserved, in syrup or as jam.

Raw or preserved. Rarely, it seems, is fruit which is in season baked, and I have to admit that at first I was disappointed that a *torta alle ciliegie* or *torta all'albicocca* hereabouts is not a pastry tart overflowing with oven-baked cherries, their almondy stones still inside, or apricot halves, their sugars caramelized by the heat of the oven – the kind of dessert I have so enjoyed in France.

Instead, such tarts are what I, raised on British cuisine, would describe as a jam tart – *torta alle ciliegie* might translate as 'cherry tart', but it is in fact pastry slicked with cherry jam. *Torta all'albicocca* is an apricot-jam tart.

I've come to the conclusion that this is a factor of the Campomelano *cucina* born of the frugality of *cucina povera*. Because if you wanted to eat fruit whole and in season you could eat it straight from the tree; why use up eggs, flour and sugar on a fruit which Nature serves you ready to eat, when these ingredients and the wood needed to cook them can be put to other uses? But if the boughs sigh with their seasonal burden of figs or pears, too many to eat just now, good sense and thrift dictate that they should be preserved, stacked in the *cantina* and savoured whenever you wish.

Of course there's another fruit which is preserved here not out of necessity or frugality but on purpose: *l'uva per vino*, grapes for wine.

Here *uva per vino* is grown chiefly for home consumption rather than for commercial reasons, but the *vinificazione*, the wine-making, is no less serious for that. For weeks now, defining the moment of the *vendemmia*, the harvest, has been the question on everyone's lips: *presto, presto*, everyone is saying – it's early this year, because the summer was unusually hot and dry. The timing of the harvest is crucial: the grapes must be plucked when they are perfectly ripe, not overripe, to ensure the correct balance of sugar and acidity, depending on what taste the wine-maker is aiming for.

Uno di questi giorni, people tell me – any day now. I've been waiting for this moment all year, charting the slow progress of the wine daily as I whizz past the flat walls of upright vines which rank the front yard of a house on the edge of Taverna. Every day as I've driven out of the village and then back in, I've noted the changes in the vines: the grey bareness at the start of the year, the green shoots like fairy lights in the spring sun, the rampant foliage and cascading grapes of the summer followed by the red creep of autumn on the leaves. I've never seen anyone in this front yard tending these vines, and have no idea whom they belong to, but here you only have to ask for help and it's given generously, immediately.

A few inquiries in Taverna and the next thing I know Aguillino and I are in the car then parking up beside the vines, where he introduces me to Gerolomo and his wife, Anna, who are already collecting the grapes. It's heading towards dusk, and they and a couple of friends are racing against the darkness to hand-harvest as many as possible. Yes, of course I can watch them make the wine, they say; come back in a day or so, when they should be on the way with the red. We leave them to their work.

When I return, Gerolomo shows me how they press the wine through the *torchio*, a hand-operated, wooden-barrelled press. The grapes go in whole, Gerolomo turns the handle, and the mashed fruit waterfalls out.

This is the *mosto*, he tells me, and points to huge plastic vats where mashed skin, pips, stalks and flesh are fermenting. These will be left to macerate for five or six days, the time needed, Gerolomo says, to create a red wine with a good, rich colour from the skins and a bit of tannin from the stalks, to let the sugar turn into alcohol. The *mosto* is placed in huge plastic bottles fitted with taps at the base. Every two or three days Gerolomo will open the taps and let the *mosto* solids filter out, finally putting the remaining juices into a demijohn until the spring, when the wine will be bottled. It all seems so incredibly simple, but then Nature, left to its own devices, needs only the slightest helping hand.

Gerolomo hands me a glass of last year's white – it's light and fruity and tastes simply of grapes, nothing like the commercial wines I grew accustomed to in the UK. But then there are no chemicals in this wine, no added yeasts, a fact, I am told, that explains why I have never ever had a hangover from Campomelano wine, no matter how many glasses I have enjoyed over endless lunches.

As I leave, Gerolomo snips me bunch after bunch of white grapes from his pergola, good as *uva da tavola*, he tells me, handing me a bottle of last year's white from the shelf. The same grapes, from the same vine: some fresh for the moment, some conserved for the *cantina*.

Back home I have a kitchen full of fresh grapes – too many for the table. Some will have to be preserved. So I pick up my wicker basket and slip out to the garden to where the green figs have already begun to splatter to the ground. When I raise my hand to the green-leafy bough, barely do my fingers cup the sticky under-belly of the fruit than it falls into my grasp. The fig is so packed with sugary ripeness that the skin splits at my touch, a single drop of syrupy richness oozing out of the flesh, glistening in the evening sun, even before I bite into it.

In the kitchen I peel the figs and slice them in half, pluck the grapes from the vine stalk one by one, heat them in a pan and add sugar to turn them into jam. Soon after, it's in the jars, ready for my in-house *cantina*. The *cantina* still houses jars of *carciofini sott'olio*, the first crop I preserved here in spring, after 'Pina showed me how, and a little jar of *amarena* jam, made after an afternoon stoning the sour cherries under the pergola with Pasqualina, Assunta and Amalia. *La bottiglia*, which Theodora helped me make, and a jar of dried chillies Maria gave me. And bottles of olive oil from the groves of my friends Antonio and Nina. *Tutta roba nostra*, all our own things.

After a simple dinner of fresh eggs fried in olive oil and scat-tered with *peperoncino* and a couple of slices of Leana's freshly baked bread, I eat *uva fragola* as my fruit course, just as Pasqualina said I should. I savour the strawberry secret that lies within these grapes, knowing that soon they will be gone, not to be had for another year. But that when the mood takes me, and I want the scent of sunshine on the vine, a memory of an autumn's day making wine, I can reach into my *cantina* and enjoy these *uva fragola*. The vines will be leafless and grey, the fig tree a black etching against the winter rain, but their fruit will be vital and sun-splashed on my plate.

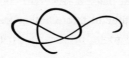

Marmellata di uva fragola e fichi –
Strawberry grape and fig jam

Here figs are considered ready to eat when they are so ripe
that they drop into your hand as you shake the bough; this
moment usually arrives around the end of September or
start of October. The *uva fragola* are ready when their skins
explode to the touch. This is the point at which they are
considered at their best for turning into jam because they
are rich in sugar, which will ensure the jam is sweet and
help the preserving process. You will require a large, deep,
heavy-based pan for this recipe, and glass preserving jars.
Use the jam to create a typical Campodimele jam *torta* with
the same pastry base as that in the recipe for *crostata
all'amarena* on page 190.

500g (1lb) organic uva fragola
500g (1lb) ripe figs – green or black
1kg (2lb) sugar
Three 350ml (12fl oz) glass jars with screw lids

Wash the fruit thoroughly. Peel the outer skin from the figs
then slice them in half and place them in the pan with the
grapes. Heat the fruit over a low flame for around half an
hour, stirring frequently to ensure its sugars don't stick to
the bottom of the pan and burn.

While the fruit is cooking, thoroughly sterilize the jars
(see page 188) and place a saucer to cool in the freezer –
this will be used later to test whether the jam has reached
setting point.

When the grapes and figs have cooked for around half an hour, pass them through a sieve or a food mill to get rid of the skins and stones.

Put the fruit back in the pan and gradually add the sugar, stirring well between each addition to ensure the sugar dissolves quickly.

Cook the jam on a low heat for a further forty minutes or so, until it starts to bubble.

To test if the jam has reached setting point, place a teaspoon of the jam onto the saucer that has been in the freezer – tilt the saucer, and if the jam clings to it and wrinkles on top, it is ready to put in jars. If this does not happen, continue boiling, replace the saucer in the freezer, and test again in a few minutes. Continue testing until the jam is ready to bottle.

Once it is ready, place it immediately in the sterilized jars and seal with screw-top lids. Jam containing equal proportions of sugar and fruit should keep for up to a year in a cool, dark place.

Makes about three 350ml (12fl oz) jars of jam.

Fragole al limone − Strawberries marinated in lemon syrup

1 kg (2lb) strawberries − wild, if available
100g (3½oz) caster sugar
Juice of a lemon − or more, according to taste
500ml (1 pint) boiling water

Wash the strawberries and slice into halves or quarters depending on their size.

Mix the sugar with the juice of a lemon and the boiling water until the sugar dissolves to create a syrup, adding more lemon juice if preferred.

Add the strawberries to the syrup and mix gently, ensuring all the fruit is covered.

Allow to marinate at room temperature for at least an hour before serving.

Serves four.

Focaccia ripiena di fichi e mozzarella –
Focaccia stuffed with figs and mozzarella

This might seem an unusual combination, but it is delicious providing the figs are super-sweet and the mozzarella same-day fresh. This cheese is very moist, so wipe away excess liquid and eat immediately to prevent the bread from going soggy. For another variation, substitute the figs with four or five slices of prosciutto cut into small pieces for ease of eating.

One large focaccia – preferably without herbs on top
Two fresh balls of mozzarella di bufala
Four ripe figs

Slice the focaccia horizontally.

Slice the mozzarella and gently pat away excess water with kitchen paper.

Peel and slice the figs horizontally, discarding the very tops and bottoms.

Layer the figs on the base of the focaccia, cover with a layer of mozzarella, and place the top layer of focaccia on top. Cut the focaccia into four wedges and eat immediately.

Makes four sandwiches, or sixteen mini-sandwiches suitable as antipasti.

Fichi secchi – Dried figs

Once upon a time, I am told, it was very common to see figs laid out to dry in the sun in Campodimele, but this meant being available to whip the fruit indoors should there be an unexpected shower. These days, those who wish to preserve figs tend to use the oven.

About twenty ripe figs, of even size

Preheat the oven to 160°C/320°F/Gas Mark 3 for around twenty minutes.

Wash and dry the figs then slice in half lengthways and place on a shallow baking tray in the oven, skin side down.

Leave the figs until they have dried out – this will take several hours and depend on the size and liquid content of the fruit.

Once the figs are dried out, allow them to cool on wire racks then store in airtight containers – they should last several weeks if stored in a cool place.

Home is the Hunter

It's *furbo*, the wild boar – crafty. Anyone will tell you so.

In the hot months, when boar hunting is banned, they raid the village by night: flattening fields of wheat as they go, devouring maize cobs on the plant; trampling the *orti* as they snuffle and snaffle their midnight feasts of the ripest foods. Then they steal back into the mountains like the brigands they are, as the first sunlight betrays their crimes.

By the light of the summer moon you can catch little gangs of wild boar roaming the village roads, as if they know the hunting season is closed. One morning in July, my friend Bruno and I even met one trotting along Taverna's main street. Dark brown coat, barrel-belly, white fangs, he'd the air of an animal cocking a snook at the village men taking breakfast at Maurizio's bar.

But come the cold season, when the huntsmen dust down their guns, these wild pigs seem to know to make themselves scarce.

They no longer linger in the oak groves of the lower slopes, which are their summer haunts. Instead they cross the invisible border that curls through the Aurunci Mountains National Park, separating the territory where hunting is permitted from those areas where it is not. Just a day or two of gunshot splitting the still mountain air and the boar are off, I'm told, to the safety of the grounds out-of-bounds to hunters.

Although even during the months of *la caccia*, the hunt, they might venture down to the village after sundown, to snaffle a few winter greens, because shooting is forbidden once darkness falls, and it's clear they have a feel for the rules.

'They sleep for much of the day then rise at dusk and go out to look for food,' Italo explains, and I have an image of these wild pigs waking with *l'imbrunire*, nightfall, and heading off for their nocturnal breakfast. 'Then they come back up the mountain and find a nice warm spot in the sun, and they sleep.' It's not so much the fact that they are *furbi*, Italo says. 'They are just as intelligent as you and me.'

Maybe this is one of the keys to the game, one of the thrills of this sport, I think. Because *la caccia* is hardly a chase if the prey is too easy to catch. Boar and hares and the songbirds of these mountains were once an essential part of *cucina povera*, free food at a time when meat was a rare luxury. Today most people here can afford to raise their own livestock or buy meat whenever they wish – but wild boar meat is not to be bought, nor are the leaping hares or the mountain thrushes. Round here you hunt your game, or you don't get to eat it at home.

Hunting is a cold-season sport. The first rounds of rifle fire rattle round the arena of the valley in October, when the season for leaping hare begins. November brings the start of the wild boar season. The clientele at the piazza's Moonlight Café will pause and cock their heads, like dogs catching a footstep on the wind, and debate how well the hunting is going this season. Few shots are taken as a poor sign, a larder that will be short on game. Many rounds might be toasted with a thimbleful of grappa. Of course, whether the gunfire will translate into *lepre alla cacciatora*, roast hunter's hare, or *salsiccia di cinghiale*, wild boar sausage, depends on how *furbi* the animals are.

The hunting day starts early, because the autumn and winter days are short and the weather often bad, and by the end of January the season will be closed.

The hunters rise before dawn and gather at Maurizio's bar just as daylight breaks. Despite the early hour, the shivering cold, there's an air of festivity, and I am reminded that as well as sport, as well as food, the hunt represents a key part of the social and cultural fabric of Campodimele. It's a chance for those who live in the more isolated dwellings scattered across the mountainside to catch up with friends. And it's a moment when those who no longer earn their main livelihood from the land can reconnect with the rural rituals on which so many generations of their families once depended.

We fuel up on creamy cappuccinos and feathery *cornetti*, the Italian croissants that are drier, less buttery, than their French counterparts. Outside the bar the sky is flat, grey, marbled with smoky black clouds, but we can already hear the dogs barking somewhere and so we head off into the hills, the huntsmen garbed in green combat fatigues and bright orange gilets to ensure they don't get caught in crossfire. Me, in my oh-so-English Barbour and walking boots, wondering if a *cinghiale* will wander my way.

Italo and I take our place in the *ferro di cavallo*, the horseshoe formation in which the huntsmen string out, curving through the mountains behind the village. With luck there will be wild boar who bedded down within the hunting territories as dawn broke this morning, or who have straggled on their return from midnight raids, or who simply haven't sussed out the dangerous ground from the place the hunters can't go. There's the occasional yelping of the dogs, who seem to have found a scent, but then nothing to suggest a kill. 'When it's damp, like this, the dogs can't catch much scent,' Italo shrugs.

We wait and wait, amid the etched outlines of the oak trees on whose acorns the *cinghiali* gorge and which help give their flesh its earthy, gamey note. But the wind brings us nothing but the steady sighs of its own damp breath and that of the naked, shivering trees.

And then a gunshot, two, their echoes rippling through the folds of the mountains like a round of applause. But it's too far away to know if there's a kill. We'll find out when we head back to the Moonlight Café for a mid-morning espresso. 'Pina will have the news. Or maybe some successful hunters will be there. You can so often spot someone who has brought a wild boar in. He's the one with the animated smile, the louder laugh, the one offering grappa shots all round. The one who is thrilled to be alive. There is something about hunting which connects with the very soul of men, I believe. Perhaps it truly does stir those instincts of humankind's primeval past. I have city friends who could never condone hunting. But here, where Nature never lets you forget that death is an integral part of life, hunting for food emerges as the most natural occupation of all.

The huntsmen have been kind enough to let me be their guest on a number of days, and though I have never seen an animal shot, I have seen the joy with which such a day ends.

Earlier in the year, I was drinking espresso at the Moonlight Café when Roberto, one of the younger huntsmen, rang my mobile. He and his brother Francesco run Lo Stuzzichino, a restaurant-pizzeria in Taverna which attracts clientele from all the surrounding cities thanks to the quality of Francesco's cooking and its meat. For those unable to hunt their own, Lo Stuzzichino is a first destination to enjoy dishes made with wild boar.

Two boar had been killed, Roberto told me. His father, Fiore, would be butchering them soon. I could watch if I wished to.

So I did. They call Fiore '*il maestro*', 'the master', and watching him, it is easy to see why. The dead pigs hung by their back hooves from a stick suspended from the ceiling in Italo's *cantina*. With a scalpel-sharp knife, Fiore cut a circular incision around one of the boar's rear ankles then stripped back the hide, little by little, to reveal the flesh beneath. Then, seizing a machete, he sliced the torso open from head to tail, and removed the heart, lungs and liver to be washed and chopped and seasoned and formed into the prized *salsicce di fegato*, liver sausage of wild boar. Fiore worked quietly, quickly, with an intense concentration, perhaps because no meat is more prized around here.

The numbers explain why. An average-sized animal might weigh 150 kilos, with around 30 per cent of that suitable as meat for the pot. Over a season, the hunt might take around sixty *cinghiali*. Or perhaps fewer. The kill is divided equally among the total number of hunters who were on the hill on the given day – perhaps forty, possibly more. But there is more than scarcity and delicious taste to the popularity of wild boar, I think. Wild game comes to your table with a history: memories of how it was hunted, recollections of the day on the hill, time spent with friends.

So it is treasured like rubies: cooked gently with white wine, herbs, a little tomato *sugo*. Maybe eaten straightaway. But often it will be frozen and saved for celebratory days – 25 December or *Capo d'Anno*, New Year. It will be served with *pappardelle*, thick, flat ribbons of *pasta all'uovo*. Or perhaps with polenta, though this is not really polenta country, I am told, the corn grown here usually being saved to feed the hens.

In the summer, boar is served out of season at *La Festa del Cacciatore*, the Hunter's Festival, and people flock to the village to taste it. It's served with polenta then, the fine ground corn poured into a huge vat on the street in Taverna, the hunters taking turns to stir it with a wooden paddle over an open flame. I can't help feeling there is a little irony in this: is the polenta ground from cobs from the same fields the crafty boar so love to raid in the summertime?

I remember bidding goodnight to Italo and Fiore that winter's eve. Darkness lay like a sheet across the sky. The moon was hiding behind a cloud. Light blazed from Maurizio's bar, and laughter and camaraderie bubbled out onto the street. The village still buzzed with the success of the hunt.

But the scent of wood-smoke was growing stronger on the air, calling the hunters home to dinner by log fires. And the guns were down for another day. That day's wild boar were not yet ready to eat, but their stories would help the hunters savour the evening meal. There would be accounts of the day on the hill, where the boar were found. How *il cinghiale furbo* had been outwitted, just this once.

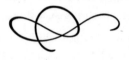

Antipasti di montagna – Antipasti of the mountains

Wild game sausage, air-dried *salsicce*, goat's cheese, olives – these are the foods of the mountains, brought together in a single plate of appetizers to serve ahead of the *primo* course of pasta.

Selection of sliced salumi, such as wild boar sausage, sweet pork sausage (without hot chilli pepper), spicy pork sausage (with hot chilli pepper) and prosciutto; aim for about six slices of meat per diner

Selection of fresh and matured mountain cheeses, such as formaggio di capra (fresh goat's cheese), formaggio di pecora (fresh sheep's cheese) and Pecorino Romano (matured sheep's cheese), sliced finely; aim for about 100g (4oz) cheese per diner

Handful of Italian olives marinated in olive oil, crushed garlic cloves, wild fennel seeds and crushed dried hot chilli pepper for at least two hours (see page 22)

Handful of olive semplici – simple olives, prepared only in their conserving brine

Arrange the finely sliced *salumi*, cheese and olives on a large serving plate just a few minutes before serving, to prevent the food drying out. Serve immediately.

Lepre alla cacciatora – Hunter's hare

Hares just a few months old – known as leverets – are the best for roasting. They can be difficult to procure, but this recipe works equally well with rabbit.

One young hare, cut into pieces, or rabbit
One large golden onion, roughly sliced
Four large cloves of garlic, squashed against the side of a knife
Few sprigs of fresh rosemary, bruised to release their oils
500ml (1 pint) good dry white wine
Fine sea salt
Few splashes of extra-virgin olive oil
Handful of chopped fresh plum or cherry tomatoes (optional)

Place the hare in a large bowl along with the onion, garlic, rosemary and white wine, and leave to marinate in the fridge for around twelve hours.

Remove the hare pieces from the marinade and place in a colander to drain for around half an hour, to allow the flesh to dry out and return to room temperature.

Preheat the oven to 180°C/350°F/Gas Mark 4.

Pat the hare dry with kitchen paper, and season with a few pinches of sea salt, to taste.

Heat the olive oil on the stove in a flameproof roasting tin, and place the hare in it. Cook for a few minutes on each side, until golden brown all over.

Next, add the onion, garlic, rosemary and white wine marinade to the roasting tin, along with the chopped tomatoes, if using. Bring gently to simmering point then immediately place the roasting tin on the middle shelf of the oven.

Cook the hare pieces for around forty-five minutes to an hour, basting them frequently with the cooking juices. Serve hot.

Serves six.

Spezzatino di cinghiale con polenta –
Wild boar stew with polenta

Instead of polenta, wild boar stew can be served with *pappardelle* ribbons (see pages 51–57).

For the stew:
1kg (2lb) wild boar shoulder, on the bone if available
Few splashes of extra-virgin olive oil
Three large cloves of garlic, roughly chopped
One large golden onion, finely sliced
One bay leaf
Sprig of fresh rosemary, bruised to release its juices
Fine sea salt
Crushed dried red chilli
Two large glasses of good dry white wine
1 litre (2 pints) conserved tomato sauce (see page 263)

For the polenta:
400g (14oz) polenta flour

Cut the wild boar into pieces about 5cm (2in) square.

Place in a large, deep pan, along with a few tablespoons of cold water, bring to the simmer, and allow the meat to cook gently for fifteen to twenty minutes, allowing the game to emit most of the strong-tasting juices.

Drain the meat, discarding the liquid.

Heat the olive oil in a large, deep pan, add the garlic, onion, bay leaf and rosemary. Fry gently for a few minutes. Add two good pinches of salt, and a pinch of chilli.

Turn up the heat then add the drained wild boar meat to the pan, and fry it for a few minutes, turning it frequently until it browns on all sides. Lower the heat and continue cooking for a further fifteen minutes or so.

Next, add the wine, and allow to cook for a few minutes until the wine has reduced by about a third.

Add the tomato sauce, return to a simmer, cover, and allow to cook gently for around an hour and a half, stirring frequently.

When the meat is tender and flakes easily against the tines of a fork, it is ready. Add extra salt to taste. It can be eaten immediately, but tastes even more delicious if left overnight – cooled, refrigerated in a covered container then gently reheated the next day.

About forty-five minutes before the stew is ready to be served, start to prepare the polenta – much commercially available polenta is quick-cook, in which case follow the instructions on the packet. If you can, buy untreated polenta flour and cook according to the instructions below.

Pour 1 litre (2 pints) of water into a large, deep pan, add two or three good pinches of sea salt, and bring to the boil. Meanwhile, keep a further half litre (1 pint) of salted water boiling in an adjacent pan, in case it is needed.

Pour the polenta into the boiling water in a slow, steady stream, stirring constantly with a long wooden spoon. The polenta will gradually thicken. Lower the heat a little, and continue stirring for forty-five minutes to an hour, until the polenta is cooked to the consistency of mashed potato. If the polenta becomes too thick, add a ladleful of water as it cooks, and mix thoroughly.

Serve immediately, along with the stew.

Serves four to six.

Spezzatino di cinghiale e lepre –
Wild boar and wild hare stew

Create this main course in the same way as for the *Spezzatino di cinghiale* (see page 300). It really is worth making this dish a day in advance of eating, to allow the flavours of the game to meld and develop.

1 kg (2lb 3oz) wild boar shoulder, on the bone if available
500g (1lb 2oz) wild hare, cut into pieces
Few splashes of extra-virgin olive oil
Three large cloves of garlic, roughly chopped
One large golden onion, finely sliced
One bay leaf
Sprig of fresh rosemary, bruised to release its juices
Fine sea salt
Crushed dried red chilli
Two large glasses of good dry white wine
1 litre (2 pints) conserved tomato sauce (see page 263)
One quantity of fresh egg pappardelle ribbons (see pages 51–57), or 400g (14oz) dried pappardelle

Follow the recipe for *Spezzatino di cinghiale*, adding the wild hare to the pan with the wild boar at the point where you are frying the boar gently in olive oil to brown it.

Serve with the *pappardelle* ribbons.

Serves four to six.

NOVEMBER

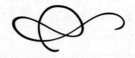

Potatoes for Gnocchi

I'm buying potatoes for gnocchi at Campodimele's open-air Wednesday market when Marietta introduces herself.

'You want the starchy potatoes if you're making gnocchi,' are her opening words. 'The older ones are the best. I'm Marietta – and you are . . .?'

It's an archetypal Italian moment. Ask a stall-holder for a kilo of aubergines and he'll inquire whether you want them for frying, roasting or preserving. Respond that you want to roast them and the *signora* next to you will advise you to scoop out the flesh, mix it with tomatoes, garlic and parsley, stuff the mixture back into the shells and bake them for half an hour. As you thank her, the lady next to her will tell you, 'No, no, no! You must add a bit of basil and pecorino too, and cook them for at least forty-five minutes, along with plenty of olive oil.' That's when the argument starts. And before you know it, the whole queue is joining in.

I love these moments, which happen daily here. In Campodimele there is no concept of nipping out for ten minutes to grab what you want to make for lunch. An intended quick trip to the market invariably turns into an impromptu cookery class: a stall-holder recommending that cherries for jam will be better next week, because sun is forecast; a friend reporting that the first broad beans of the season have arrived, so be sure to buy some pecorino to eat with them; strangers arguing over how you should cook the *broc-coletti* you are buying for lunch. Chances are you will find yourself invited to take an aperitif at the Moonlight Café before being invited to lunch, so you can watch the disputed dish being prepared with your own eyes.

So it's nothing out of the ordinary to find Marietta offering me unsolicited advice and urging me to pop round to her home for a gnocchi-making demonstration.

What does surprise me, when I take up this invitation one chilly afternoon, is the breathtaking force with which she pummels the gnocchi paste and the swiftness with which they are made. Not because I've always understood gnocchi-making to require the gentlest of hands and a lot of time. But because I can't imagine where she gets such strength to knead the gnocchi dough, and such speed in serving them up.

Marietta is eighty-nine and lives alone in her centuries-old stone house on one of the winding cobbled streets that follow the curve of Campodimele's medieval walls. Her kitchen is tiny – the size of a large cupboard – but perfectly arranged and stocked so that she has everything to hand when I drop by to discuss when we might make the said gnocchi. '*Ora!*' she insists, unfazed by the notion of improvising a cookery class on the spur of the moment. 'Now!' She is already spooning coffee into the aluminium Moka pot and placing it on the stove: hospitality is, it seems, the first duty for every Italian.

The word *gnocchi*, which translates as 'little lumps', is used to describe a range of dumplings made from varying ingredients. In some parts of Italy, eggs are added to the paste, to make what is known as *gnocchi alla parigina* – Parisian gnocchi – but in Campodimele, they are traditionally made with just flour, potatoes and a pinch of salt. When times were leaner, eggs could be put to better use in other dishes.

Despite their minimal ingredients, gnocchi are considered a bothersome and time-consuming dish to prepare by many of the Campomelani with whom I have discussed them. But in Marietta's hands this is not the case. By the time the espresso is in the tiny china cups, the potatoes are already boiling, still in their skins, to ensure they do not become waterlogged. Marietta places a large wooden workboard on the table beneath her living-room window, half empties a bag of flour onto it and scatters a pinch of salt on top. The boiled potatoes are barely out of the water and she is slipping off their skins and squashing them through a potato ricer so that they wriggle onto the flour like vermicelli. Now she is working the potatoes into the flour, first with one hand then with two hands, moulding the mixture into a creamy dough. And now she's hammering it: her back bent over the work surface, shoulders tense, the muscles in her aged arms rippling as she shoves the heels of both hands into the paste. She works with the vigour and vitality of a pugilist.

'You have to work with the dough while it's hot!' she says, as if racing against herself. Without pause she divides the dough into sections, rolls each piece into a long sausage shape then slices each one into pieces no bigger than a thumbnail. She curls the little bits of dough against the tines of a fork, creating the indentations where the tomato sauce will settle.

At some point amid all this activity she has put a pan of salted water on to boil, and in go the gnocchi. They sink like little submarines and a minute or so later shoot back to the surface: they are ready. Marietta skims the cooked gnocchi into bowls and splashes a spoonful or two of hot tomato sauce over them – sauce she made last summer.

The gnocchi are like plumped-up cushions, both firm and yield-ing, with a delicate potato taste. They slide down with a satisfying warmth, the sauce a slick of summer out of season. This is a substan-tial dish, usually served as a *primo* in place of pasta. As I wave goodbye to Marietta, I wonder again how, in her ninth decade, she maintains the strength to pummel the gnocchi paste that way. When I ask her this, she simply shrugs.

I discover the answer to my question some time later. If you happen by Campodimele in the early evening, you will find yourself invited by the bells to attend Mass at San Michele Arcangelo, the church of St Michael the Archangel. The bells in its tower ring three times: thirty minutes before Mass begins, fifteen minutes later, then a third time, as Mass is about to start.

I slipped into church after the third call to prayer one evening just in time to spot an elderly lady emerging from a door by the north window. She genuflected before the altar then took a seat in the front pew, as Don Leone, who was parish priest when I first arrived in Campodimele, commenced Mass.

The elderly lady was the *campanara*, the official bell-ringer of the church, with thirty years' experience of calling worshippers to Mass several times a week. Hauling the three ropes of the ancient brass bells, her role was to signal the religious rituals of village life. When babies are baptized and when couples wed, the *campanara* peals out the joy of new beginnings. When a villager has passed away, the mountain air is stilled by the solemn toll of the mourning bells.

The *campanara* that evening was Marietta, who found me buying potatoes in the marketplace and invited me home to show me how gnocchi are made.

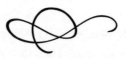

Gnocchi al ragù –
Gnocchi with ragù of pork, beef and pork sausage

This is one of the most popular ways of serving gnocchi in Campodimele, and is a delicious, satisfying supper on a cold evening.

One quantity pork, beef and pork sausage ragù (see page 51)
One quantity potato gnocchi (see page 310)
100g (4oz) freshly grated Parmigiano-Reggiano, if desired

Make the *ragù*, and, about thirty minutes before it is ready to serve, place it on a low simmer while you make the gnocchi.

Make one quantity of potato gnocchi according to the instructions on page 310–11, and when they are cooked, use a slotted spoon to skim them into warm serving bowls.

Remove the *ragù* from the heat and tilt the pan, carefully ladling out the liquidy sauce spoon it over the gnocchi. Scatter over the grated Parmesan, if using.

For a hearty one-plate meal, serve chunks of the pork, beef and sausage in the same bowl as the gnocchi. Alternatively serve as a second course, with a *contorno* of leafy greens.

Serves four.

Gnocchi di patate con sugo di pomodoro –
Potato gnocchi with home-made tomato sauce

Gnocchi-making is not an exact science: the amount of flour you require will depend on how much the potatoes absorb, and this is one of those dishes for which a trial-and-error philosophy must be adopted! Try to use potatoes of the same size so they all cook at the same time, and don't allow the dough to go cold. Despite Marietta's approach, as a general rule work the dough lightly, to avoid it becoming too soft and requiring the addition of extra flour.

500g (1lb 2oz) potatoes suitable for boiling – Desiree are perfect for this recipe
Fine sea salt
450g (1lb) '00' Doppio Zero flour or plain flour, sieved
500ml (1 pint) conserved tomato sauce (see page 263)
Fresh basil to garnish, if desired
100g (3½oz) freshly grated Parmigiano-Reggiano, if desired

Scrub the potatoes clean, and, leaving the skins on, place them in a pan of cold water and bring to the boil. Boil until tender then drain.

Place a large, wide pan of salted water on the stove – this is to cook the gnocchi once they are formed, and the wider the surface area the more cooking space the dumplings will have.

When the potatoes are cool enough to handle – but still hot – tear away the skins and discard them.

Sieve about 400g (14oz) of the flour onto a large, clean

work surface, and quickly run the potatoes through a potato ricer and straight onto the flour. Work the flour into the potatoes until you have a soft, smooth dough that is just slightly sticky. If it feels very sticky, gradually work in more of the remaining 50g (2oz) of flour until the consistency feels smooth and pliable, but not sticky.

Flour your work surface then divide the dough into four parts. Roll each piece of dough into a long sausage shape just over 2cm (1in) thick. Slice each sausage into small pieces around 2cm (1in) long to create the gnocchi.

Now you need to shape the gnocchi into small curls and create grooves on their surfaces to help them hold the sauce. To do this, hold each gnocchi against the inner curve of a fork with one finger then gently roll it down the tines.

Now put the tomato sauce on to heat so it is ready to serve when the gnocchi are cooked.

Drop the gnocchi into the pan – they will sink, but when they return to the surface allow them to cook for around fifteen seconds more then remove them with a slotted spoon and place in warm bowls. Spoon the tomato sauce over them, and scatter the basil and grated Parmesan on top, if using.

Serves four.

Gnocchi al pesto – Gnocchi with pesto sauce

Pesto is not traditional to Campodimele, but – like other recipes from far-flung parts of Italy – it has found its way up the mountain road and makes a delicious dish in summer, when fresh basil is in abundance. This recipe uses pecorino, which is local to Campodimele, instead of the *Parmigiano-Reggiano* traditionally used in pesto sauce.

For the pesto:
One clove of garlic
Large handful of fresh basil leaves
Handful of pine nuts
Fine sea salt
Few good splashes of extra-virgin olive oil
About 200g (7oz) freshly grated Pecorino Romano

For the gnocchi:
One quantity, made to the recipe on page 310

To make the pesto, crush the garlic clove, basil, pine nuts and a pinch of salt to a paste using a pestle and mortar. Stir in the olive oil and cheese, mixing thoroughly. Pecorino is quite salty, but add a little more, if desired.

When the gnocchi are ready, drain and serve immediately, bathed in the pesto.

Serves four.

The Wood-Fired Oven

For me, this is the scent of the mountains: wood-smoke wafting on a summer's dawn, its bosky breath the base note of a winter's eve.

Every place has its own aroma, its signature scents. In nearby Fondi, you're seduced by Italian city smells: the bitterness of coffee on a crisp winter morning, slicing the buttery sweetness of the *pasticceria*; the breath of orange blossom on a balmy spring night, whispering on your skin like a lover's sigh. Heading home from Fondi, via the higgledy-piggledy hilltown of Lenola, you might catch the smell of wet grass on a summer meadow, or the whiff of animal feed on an autumn field.

But as you climb towards the mountains, it's the wood-smoke that welcomes you. You'll catch its scent before you pass the road-side farmhouse where the branches are burning in winter grates. Or smell it mingling with home-raised goat meat sizzling on a charcoal grill. In the winter you notice it more, but it's there in the summer too, along with the woodpiles stacked against house walls, and the women balancing bundles of branches on their heads. Because these are the branches that fuel the *forno a legna* in which bread and pizza are baked.

Luisa emerges through a mist of flour, her blue eyes blinking away the swirling motes. She's been working the bread for fifteen minutes, she says, indicating the pizza dough in which her hands are buried. Another thirty or so and it will be done.

It's her home-grown flour in the *maniella*. And a home-made *lievito madre*. I love the tales of leavening I hear in Campodimele – the thought that the *lievito madre* lives on in the bread Luisa is making today. But I am disappointed at the youth of this one: Luisa says she created it just ten years ago. My friends Maria and Theodora employ *lieviti* started by women in their families in generations long past.

Last night Luisa mixed the *lievito madre* with tepid water to allow it to ferment further. Rising in the early hours, she poured the watery leavening into a well in her home-grown flour and, handful by handful, drew the flour from the edges into the moist centre. Now she has worked all the flour into the dough and is kneading it, pounding it, and yes, she says, it is terribly hard work, especially a batch this big. She is making fifteen pizzas for a family celebration this weekend. But she wouldn't dream of using a kneading machine, she adds, because it might overwork the dough, and you need to mould it *piano, piano* – gently, gently – if you want the bread to retain its freshness for several days. I tell her about the home bread-making machines that enjoyed a recent vogue in the UK: counter-top mixers-cum-ovens which require nothing more of the cook than to measure the ingredients out and flick the switch. She smiles a wry smile, and as she lowers her eyes to her working hands I see the magic of her craft: the dough heaving beneath her fingers like fresh-spewn lava, as if to remind us that this simple mix of flour and salt and water is a living, breathing thing. Then Luisa wraps up the dough-filled *maniella* like a baby, in a snow-white sheet and woollen blankets, and leaves it to grow.

Luisa's house is modern, perhaps only a decade old, but the north-east corner of her kitchen could have been created centuries ago. In it are stacked tools with handles a metre, maybe 2 metres, long: a paddle with a perfectly flat face; a broom with a short and wispy tail; another tipped with long dried grass dusted with swept-up flour. Beside them the whitewashed wall curves to a lip, and above this rests a little metal shield complete with curlicue handle, flush with the wall. Luisa sweeps the shield away to expose a gaping mouth in the wall and, like the breath of a dragon, out comes the heat from the orange inferno of her wood-fired oven.

'*Acero, quercia*' – maple, oak. Louisa stokes the branches, which must burn to charcoal before the pizza can bake in their heat. She chooses these woods for the perfume they emit as they burn, and it is their scent, the sweet smokiness of charred wood, that will seep into the bread as it bakes, creating the incomparable taste of *pane al forno a legna*, bread baked in a wood-fired oven.

The pizza dough *sta crescendo*, is rising. The wood is reducing to *brace*. This is the pause in which to prepare the vegetables that will top and fill the pizza. Luisa has three favourite types of pizza – *rossa*, red, which is Italian shorthand for any dish whose signature note is tomatoes; *con patate*, wafer-thin discs of potatoes scattered with rosemary and freshly chopped red chilli pepper; and *con le verdure*, green leafy vegetables boiled, strained, perhaps mixed with a few chopped olives and used as the filling for a lidded pizza that resembles a pie or tart.

Luisa slices tiny cherry tomatoes in half, and leaves them to marinate in a bowl with a few basil leaves and roughly chopped fresh garlic. She cuts the potatoes with a serrated knife so they will bake to a golden crisp in the oven. The *verdura* today is *cicoria*, the green, leafy vegetable that bears no resemblance to the pale green endive British people describe as chicory. In season, all the vegetables come from Luisa's *orto*, meaning that every part of her pizzas is home-produced, just like the olive oil with which she is greasing the metal tins in which her pizzas will be baked.

It takes about two hours for the dough to rise, though this always depends on the humidity outdoors and the warmth of the kitchen – Nature only knows why. Luisa unwraps the *maniella* to reveal the risen dough, huge and smooth as the side of a scalded pig, and as she rips away a handful you can see that inside it is bubbling with lazy life.

She works quickly now, pulling and stretching a piece of dough between her hands then moulding it to cover the base of a circular baking tin. Then she spreads it with a tangle of leafy greens, places another disc of dough on top and squidges the edges together to create a *pizza ripiena*, a filled pizza, a dish found often around here. Her pizza *rossa* and pizza *con patate* are the classic flatbreads, a single layer topped with the red, green and white of tomato, basil and garlic or chilli pepper, rosemary and potato.

With a sweep of her arm she opens the little door on her *forno a legna* to find the burnt-down *brace* glowing like amber jewels. Then one by one she places the pizzas on her flat-faced paddle and feeds them into the mouth of the waiting oven, straight onto its stony floor, before sealing it up again.

It takes just minutes, ten, maybe twelve, and even then there is just the faintest hint of baking bread permeating the kitchen air. When Luisa opens up the oven, for a moment there is nothing but heat, and the sweet smell of new-baked dough and the scrape of the paddle on the oven floor as she lifts out the pizzas. They emerge hissing and spitting, the potatoes crisp and curly, the tomatoes collapsed and running with juice, the bread bases swollen and deep. It's *un altro gusto*, a better taste, compared to the pizza I know. The bread is light with air, rich with oil, and in each bite you catch the faintest breath of the smoky branches by which it was cooked. Perfect, in its simplicity.

I'm driving home from Luisa's house in Taverna, up the skinny backroads that straggle behind the village. Skirting fields where wheat whispers in summer breezes, but which lay bare in the winter months. Past the empty and broken-down stone house whose windows no longer see. And the still-under-construction villa that is probably waiting for a new groom and his bride. One property no longer inhabited, the other yet to be lived in, but both, I suspect, reserving a place for a wood-fired oven. Neither dwelling can be burning wood today, and along this road there are no other houses. But still I can smell wood-smoke. It might be floating down from Campodimele's *centro storico*, or up from Pozzo della Valle, the shepherds' settlement, whose name means 'Well in the Valley'. I can't tell, because the wind is blowing every way today. But as the road carries me up towards the oak groves where the wood-smoke begins, I know this is the scent that tells me I'm home.

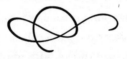

Pizza rossa – Tomato pizza

One batch of bread dough (see page 229)
1kg (2lb 3oz) cherry tomatoes or baby plum tomatoes, halved
Four cloves of garlic, very finely sliced
A few fresh basil leaves, torn into small pieces
Fine sea salt
Few splashes of extra-virgin olive oil

Make the pizza dough and leave it somewhere warm to leaven for two to three hours, until it has doubled in size.

Set branches to burn in the wood-fired oven immediately, if using.

Lightly oil four round pizza pans, each of them measuring 27cm (11in) wide and 3cm (1in) deep.

Next, prepare the topping. Mix the halved tomatoes in a large bowl with the garlic, basil, a pinch of salt and a splash of olive oil, and leave to marinate for half an hour or so.

When the dough is leavened and the charcoal is ready, divide the dough into four and use it to line the pizza pans.

If using a conventional oven to cook the pizzas, preheat it now to 220°C/425°F/Gas Mark 7.

Divide the topping between the bread bases, splash with a little extra olive oil, and bake immediately in the oven for twelve to fifteen minutes – they are ready when the pizzas are risen and the edges golden and crisp.

Makes four large pizzas.

Pizza con patate, rosmarino e peperoncino —
Potato, rosemary and chilli pizza

One batch of bread dough (see page 229)
500g (1lb 2oz) waxy new potatoes, peeled and finely sliced,
*   set aside in a bowl of water*
One small sprig of fresh rosemary, shredded
Two cloves of garlic, finely sliced
Two small hot chilli peppers, finely sliced
Few splashes of extra-virgin olive oil
Fine sea salt

Make the pizza dough and leave it somewhere warm
to leaven for two to three hours.

Set branches to burn in the wood-fired oven, if using.

Lightly oil four round pizza pans, each measuring 27cm
(11in) wide and 3cm (1in) deep.

Once the charcoal is ready and the dough is leavened, divide
the dough into four, and use each quarter to line a pizza pan.

If using a conventional oven to cook the pizzas, preheat
to 220°C/425°F/Gas Mark 7 now.

Pat dry the potato slices then arrange them in slightly
overlapping concentric rings over the pizza bases.

Rub the rosemary leaves between your fingers, releasing oils. Scatter over the potatoes along with the garlic, the
chilli, a splash of olive oil and a pinch of sea salt.

Place in the oven and cook for twelve to fifteen minutes,
until the edges are crisp and golden.

Makes four large pizzas.

Pizza verde – Pizza stuffed with leafy greens

This style of *pizza ripiena* is typically filled with *verdure* and the recipe uses *cicoria,* chicory greens. Alternatively, use spinach, swiss chard or leafy turnip-top greens.

One batch of bread dough (see page 229)
1.5kg (3lb 5oz) cicoria (not Belgian endive)
Large handful of black olives, stoned and chopped
Six large garlic cloves, very roughly chopped
Few splashes of extra-virgin olive oil
Fine sea salt

Make the pizza dough and set it aside somewhere warm to leaven for two to three hours, until it doubles in size.

Now set the branches to burn, if using a wood-fired oven.

Lightly oil three round pizza pans each of them measuring 27cm (11in) wide by 3cm (1in) deep.

Prepare the chicory greens – boil for around ten minutes, drain and refresh in cold water then squeeze out every last drop of water, or the pizza dough might go soggy. Chop roughly then place in a large bowl and stir in the olives, garlic, a couple of splashes of olive oil and a pinch or two of sea salt, to taste.

Once the bread dough is leavened and the oven ready, divide the dough into three pieces.

If using a conventional oven, preheat it to 220°C/425°F/ Gas Mark 7 now.

Each piece of dough must make a base and a lid for each of the three pizzas, so, taking the first piece of dough, split it in two by a ratio of one third to two thirds. Use the larger part to line the base of the pizza tin, being sure the dough comes up the sides of the tin, overhanging by 1cm (½in) or so.

Spread a third of the greens mixture onto the pizza base.

Take the remaining third of the first piece of dough and stretch or lightly roll it into a thin circle just big enough to form a lid for the pizza. Place this over the greens then seal the lid to the base. To do this, insert the tines of a fork between the pizza-base dough and the sides of the tin, place the index finger of your other hand onto the outer edge of the pizza lid, and use the fork tines to pull the base dough up and over your finger to meet the lid, securing the two with a spearing action of the tines.

When the lid is sealed onto the base, use the fork to make several small holes across the surface of the pizza, to allow moisture to escape during cooking.

Repeat this process with the two remaining pieces of dough, to create three stuffed pizzas.

Bake the pizzas for around fifteen minutes – they will need a little longer than the classic flat pizza to ensure that the bread beneath the stuffing has cooked properly. When the tops are a deep golden brown, remove them from the oven, and, using a metal palette knife, lift the pizzas so you can see the bottoms of the bases – they are ready if they are a deep golden brown. If not, give them a few minutes more in the oven.

Makes three stuffed pizzas.

Pizza ripiena di salsiccia e broccoletti –
Pizza stuffed with pork sausage and broccoletti

The earthy winter taste of *broccoletti* is a perfect foil for the sweetness of *salsiccia*. *Broccoletti* is in season in the winter, when families here traditionally kill the family pig, and the two have, by serendipitous necessity, become a classic combination.

One batch of bread dough (see page 229)
1.5kg (3lb 5oz) broccoletti
250g (9oz) salsiccia fresca dolce – non-spicy, coarse fresh pork
*   sausage*
Few splashes of extra-virgin olive oil
One large clove of garlic, roughly chopped
Fine sea salt
Few pinches of crushed dried red chilli, if desired

Make this pizza in the same way as the *pizza verde* on page 320, but instead of the *cicoria* greens use a mixture of *broccoletti* and fresh pork sausage, made according to the instructions below.

For the stuffing, boil the *broccoletti* in a large pan of water for around ten to fifteen minutes until soft to the bite, drain and refresh in cold water then squeeze out every last drop of water, to prevent the pizza dough going soggy.

Next, roughly chop the *broccoletti* and set them aside in a large bowl.

Remove the sausage meat from the skins, roughly chop and fry for a minute or two in a splash of olive oil.

Add to the bowl of *broccoletti* along with a splash or two of olive oil, the garlic and a pinch or two of sea salt, to taste. Add a pinch or two of chilli, if you prefer. Stir gently but thoroughly, ensuring the sausage meat is well distributed. Construct the pizzas and bake them as per the instructions for *pizza verde*.

Makes three stuffed pizzas.

Calzone ripieno – Folded, stuffed pizza

One batch of bread dough (see page 229)
Few splashes of extra-virgin olive oil
One large golden onion, thinly sliced into half-moons
Four large zucchine, finely sliced into thin discs
Two large garlic cloves, roughly chopped
Large handful of fresh flat-leaf parsley, finely chopped
Three medium-sized fresh organic eggs
Handful of freshly grated Parmigiano-Reggiano or Pecorino Romano
Fine sea salt

Make the pizza dough, and then set it aside somewhere warm to leaven for two to three hours, until it has doubled its original size.

If using a wood-fired oven, set the branches to burn now.

Lightly oil two flat baking trays.

When the bread is fully leavened, if using a conventional oven, preheat it to 220°C/425°F/Gas Mark 7 now.

Heat a splash or two of olive oil in a large, deep frying pan, and sauté the onions for a minute or two over a high flame, but ensure they do not brown.

Add the *zucchine* to the pan, and continue to sauté for a minute or so more.

Add the garlic and parsley, and cook for a further minute or so, ensuring the garlic does not colour, then remove the pan from the heat.

In a large bowl, beat two of the eggs then beat in the grated cheese. Add a pinch or two of salt, if desired, but bear in mind that the cheese is already very salty.

Now tip the vegetables from the pan into the egg and cheese mixture and stir thoroughly, to ensure that all the vegetables are coated with the eggs and cheese.

Next, divide the leavened dough into six pieces and stretch, or lightly roll, each piece into a circle around 20cm (8in) in diameter.

Place equal amounts of the vegetable mixture onto the dough circles, just south of the central hemisphere line. Leave a border of dough at least 3cm (1in) deep all around.

Beat the third egg then brush the outer borders of the dough circles with it.

Now fold the top half of the dough over the bottom half which holds the vegetables, aligning the edges to create a semicircle – similar to a British pasty.

Squeeze the two layers of dough together around the edges by placing the index finger and thumb of one hand onto the edge of the dough, and the index finger of the other hand between them, and squeezing the outer two digits to crimp the dough. Repeat all around the edges of each *calzone*.

Place on the baking trays and bake for around twelve to fifteen minutes, or until the dough has risen and the *calzoni* are golden on both the top and the bottom. Eat hot or cold.

Makes six medium-sized *calzoni*.

December

A Christmas Vigil

'*Aspettiamo Gesù*,' says Theodora, embracing me into her home with a kiss on each cheek, 'we're waiting for Jesus.'

It's early evening, Christmas Eve, and Campodimele is wrapped in the ever-deepening darkness of these December nights. The blackness of winter here is overwhelming. It chases you homewards up the mountain road and swaddles you as soon as you step onto the street. It peers through the windows until you draw the shutters to close it out.

But there is light amid this darkness: in the twinkle of the festive street decorations, the glow of candlelight in the shrine to the Virgin and, on clear nights, the shy sparkle of starlight in the never-ending sky.

And there's the light that beckons you to the *presepi*, the Christmas cribs that are indeed waiting for the baby Jesus.

The *presepio* is the focal point of every home just now, perhaps the one fixture that can supplant the kitchen as the centrepoint of an Italian household. These cribs are astonishingly elaborate compared to the simple Nativity scenes I'm accustomed to, wooden models conjuring up the entire village of Bethlehem in multi-layered landscapes of houses and hostelries. Joseph and Mary are depicted perhaps once, but sometimes three times – travelling with their donkey, seeking shelter at an inn, bedded down among the cows and goats. Theodora's husband, Gigino, made their *prese-pio* with his own hands, and whenever I've entered their home these past few days I've found myself drawn to the light glowing from the stable scene. Stooping to peer closer, I find the holy couple flanked by shepherds and kings. The manger is empty, save for a smattering of golden straw.

Italians call Christmas Eve '*La Vigilia*', 'the vigil', the time of waiting. Come the evening and families gather, exchange gifts and then sit down to eat. But the spiritual significance of this evening shines through. Most people I know here are *credenti*, believers in the Christian God, and while *La Vigilia* is a moment to reunite with those you love, it's also a time to commune with things beyond this mortal coil. Above the laughter and chatter, beyond the lyrical rivers of Italian language, there's a tangible sense of private prayer, a silent anticipation, an acknowledgement of mysteries we cannot explain.

The religious nature of this *festa* is evident on the table too. *La Vigilia* is designated by the Catholic Church as a day when meat should not be eaten.

So although this is a celebratory meal, there are no antipasti of *salsicce*, no pasta slicked with rich beef *ragù*, no *secondo* of goat or chicken – the one-time luxuries of meat now traditionally eaten on *festa* days. Instead seafood and fish are served. In Campodimele this often means fresh clams and squid and prawns from the nearby coastal towns of Gaeta or Formia, and *baccalà*.

Twelve of us sit down for *La Vigilia* dinner, in the way that epitomizes the Italian relationship with food. Here are grandparents, children, grandchildren – three generations who gather with *bonomia*, an ease that highlights the way Italians love to *stare in compagnia* at the table. And there's me, a foreigner and a guest in this house in which

I have been made to feel so much at home, thanks to the legendary hospitality of these generous people, this gregarious nation, and the unlimited kindness of Gigino and Theodora.

First we eat the antipasti – green olives, rocket and Parmesan salad, *mozzarella di bufala*, aubergines and peppers which have been preserved in oil. And little pieces of pizza, the deep dough base as feather-light as an angel's wing, the tomato topping tasting of the sun.

Then the *primo* – *spaghetti alle vongole*, spaghetti with clam sauce, a favourite celebratory *primo*, the little shellfish juicy and salty in the cradles of their shells, flecked with parsley and chilli, in festive green and red.

Then more *secondi* than I have space left to taste – squid fried in batter, prawns cooked in extra-virgin olive oil, a cold salad of *baccalà* with red pepper and parsley. With *contorni* of asparagus fritters and *broccoletti* dressed in olive oil, and dishes I don't even reach for, there is so much to eat.

And then a simple green salad dressed with oil and vinegar to cleanse the palate, and platefuls of sliced raw fennel, its sweet aniseed taste preceding the fruit course, the little orange mandarins still attached to their lush green leaves, plucked from the citrus groves of Fondi this very day.

The meal lasts for hours – three, four, more, I think as the *prosecco* cork pops and the panettone, that mountain of rough sponge which is the Italian Christmas cake, is unveiled and carved.

Midnight is approaching, and while the laughter and fun could go on for hours, it's time to honour the reason for tonight's feast. So we wrap up against the dark and make our way up the hill to where the thousand-year-old walls hug Campodimele's historic heart, and slip up the cobbled lane and into the piazza, where the yellow light from the church door beckons us to Midnight Mass.

Another Christmas Day has arrived. The handshakes and kisses and greetings of 'Buon Natale!' have been exchanged. We float home through the darkness, rich with our sense of peace, to the warmth of Theodora's fireside for more *prosecco*, more panettone. In her *presepio* the light of the stable glows its welcome, and when I step closer I see that in the manger, nestling in the straw, is a porcelain baby, and that *La Vigilia* is over. In houses all over Campodimele, on this dark winter night, the Christ Child is born.

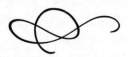

Gamberoni fritti – Fried prawns

These prawns also taste delicious if you fry a few squashed garlic cloves in the oil along with them, although I haven't met anyone in Campodimele who does this.

1kg (2lb) prawns
Handful of '00' Doppio Zero flour or plain flour
Fine sea salt
A few good splashes of extra-virgin olive oil
One lemon cut into wedges
Handful of fresh flat-leaf parsley, finely chopped

Remove the tails and claws from the prawns.

In a shallow bowl, mix the flour with a few pinches of sea salt then roll the prawns in the seasoned flour.

Heat the oil in a broad-based frying pan. When it is hot – but not too hot – add the prawns and fry for a minute or two on each side. Then remove from the pan – do not allow the prawns to colour.

Serve hot or cold, with the lemon wedges and sprinkled with the parsley, if using.

Serves six to eight as antipasti.

Spaghetti alle vongole – Spaghetti with clams

Clams should be eaten within hours of purchasing them as they do not live long. They must be thoroughly washed in lots of cold water in order to remove the sand in which they bed – asking your fishmonger to do this will save a lot of time. Before you begin cooking, remember to discard any with broken shells, or clams which do not snap shut when tapped.

2kg (4lb 6oz) small clams
400g (14oz) dried spaghetti
Four splashes of extra-virgin olive oil
Two large cloves of garlic, finely chopped
100ml (3fl oz) dry white wine
A few pinches of crushed dried red chilli
Fine sea salt
Handful of fresh flat-leaf parsley, chopped

First wash all the clams thoroughly and discard any of them that are unsuitable.

Bring a large pan of water to the boil, add a good pinch or two of salt, return to the boil and throw in the spaghetti to cook according to the instructions on the packet – usually around eight to ten minutes.

About six minutes before the spaghetti is due to be ready, heat the olive oil in a large, deep frying pan, and gently fry the garlic for around thirty seconds, making sure it does not colour – if it does, discard it and start again, as it will ruin the flavour of the dish.

Add the wine to the pan and allow to simmer for around thirty seconds then add the clams and the dried chilli. Cover the pan with a lid, and cook until the clams open – usually around five to six minutes. Add a little salt to taste.

When the spaghetti is al dente, drain it and divide into warm bowls, with a ladleful of clams on top of each plate. Sprinkle over the parsley and serve immediately.

Serves four.

Baccalà ai peperoni —
Salt cod with roasted red peppers

Like all fish and meat, dried salt cod is traditionally an expensive luxury in what is largely a vegetarian diet. Just a small piece is added to dishes like *Cicerchie in pignatta* (see page 218) to give a deliciously different flavour. You'll need to soak the cod at least a day in advance, and remember to use the finest extra-virgin olive oil for this recipe.

800g (2lb) salt cod
Two roasted red peppers, skinned (see page 275) or two red peppers
*   preserved in vinegar (see page 278)*
Few sprigs of fresh flat-leaf parsley, tough stalks removed
Handful of green olives (optional)
Few splashes of your best extra-virgin olive oil

At least twenty-four hours before you want to eat the salad, soak the dried *baccalà* in a large bowl of cold water, skin side uppermost. Change the water several times, to eliminate as much salt as possible.

Thinly slice the roasted red peppers, or slice the preserved peppers.

Drain the *baccalà* and cut into four pieces, place in a wide pan and cover with cold water. Bring the water slowly to the boil then immediately reduce the heat. Cook the salt cod on a slow simmer for around ten minutes, but no more, or it will overcook.

Drain the salt cod, pat it dry with kitchen paper, and allow it to cool fully.

Cut the salt cod into small pieces and place on a serving dish. Arrange the red peppers and parsley over it with the olives if desired, and drizzle over the extra-virgin olive oil.

Cover and set aside in a cool place for at least an hour prior to serving.

Serves four.

Torta alle mandorle – Almond cake

Panettone has become Italy's unofficial Christmas cake, filtering down from the northern region of Lombardy, where it originated, to grace festive celebrations with its domed peak and citrus-candy sponge. Aminta assures me that before beribboned boxes of panettone arrived in Campodimele, it was almond cake that was traditionally eaten here at Christmas. It works best with a few bitter almonds in the mix, but be careful – bitter almonds are poisonous unless heat-treated, so be sure to use shop-bought ones.

250g (9oz) sweet almonds, blanched
50g (2oz) bitter almonds, shop-bought
Butter, for greasing
Twelve large fresh organic eggs
12 dsstsp white caster sugar
3 dsstsp '00' Doppio Zero flour or plain white flour
2 tbsp Strega – Italian herb-infused liqueur

Three days before you wish to eat the cake, place the blanched, whole sweet and bitter almonds in a large, clear polythene bag, seal it, and lightly crush them by passing a rolling pin over them. Then tip the almonds onto a large baking tray, spread them out, and leave to air-dry in a cool, dry place for three days.

Once the almonds have completely dried out, butter a 27 by 3cm (11 by 1in) tart tin, and preheat the oven to 180°C/350°F/Gas Mark 4.

In a large bowl, beat the eggs along with the sugar until they start to form soft peaks.

Sieve the flour over the eggs, gently folding it in with a spatula as you go – don't overwork, or you will eliminate too much air.

Now add the air-dried almonds and the Strega, and mix them in well.

Tip the cake mixture into the buttered tin, spread it evenly over the base of the tin, and bake in the oven for around half an hour, until the mixture is lightly golden on top.

Serves eight to ten.

New Year

And now the year is dying. Or is it?

New Year's Eve on the calendar has the look of a literal end, but it's only a man-made measure, after all.

This one dawns with a warmth that whispers of spring mornings, a sun yellow with the promise of summer days.

And although one year is about to meet the next, you sense that here, where Nature's voice is easily heard, there aren't really endings at all. Just a continuum, and beginnings.

The farming year hasn't stopped, it's simply slowed down. The fields recline in empty blackness, and the vines have shrunk to silver fretwork on their frames. But even on the coldest, wettest days, for some things the moment is now. The olive harvest began a couple of weeks ago and it will continue into the New Year. And the goats will carry their kids through to January before bearing them in the spring.

As the clock strikes midnight tonight, the page will flip on the linear map we make of the Sun, the Moon and the Earth. But the circle of Nature will spool unbroken into the future, and you sense that in every moment here.

Capo d'Anno, the top of the year – not a death, but a birth.

So burn branches until they crumble to charcoal, to grill

home-raised lamb with winter herbs. Simmer wild boar stew and roast some hare, if your menfolk have been hunting on the hill. And raid the *cantina* for the fruits of the *orto* you have conserved these twelve months past.

New Year's Eve gathers the riches of the year's harvests at a single meal, and as heads bow for the prayer of grace, thanks are given for the plenty that has gone before. May the next year be so full of fortune, is the supplication. And as religion and superstition sit comfortably side by side here, this wish is reflected on the dinner plate too.

'*Lenticchie, per fortuna*,' says Adalgesia, indicating a pan of little green pulses on the stove – lentils, for luck. Perhaps because they are round, like coins, so symbolizing the wished-for wealth of the year to come, though nobody knows for sure.

Lenticchie con cotechino, lentils and pig's-snout sausage, is a classic *Capo d'Anno* dish in Italy and, in Campodimele, a combination of the new and the old. Lentils are not a crop typical to these mountains and must have filtered down from the plains of the north in the easier post-war years, because good things are always welcome here, and pulses a key part of the diet. Those who raise a family pig can make the thick pink sausage of *cotechino* from its snout.

We're in the kitchen of Adalgesia's son, Pasquale, and his wife, Rosana, my friend and an English teacher at a nearby school. They live in Taverna. The room has that energy which inhabits all Italian kitchens during preparations for a *festa*. Heat, steam, bubbling, hissing. Urgency tempered with experienced calm. Adalgesia and Rosana have been cooking all afternoon, and now we are washing and drying pans and pots so that more dishes can be prepared.

The table is always rich in Campodimele, even if much of the food derives from *cucina povera*. Tonight it is richer than most.

The feast is replete with fish and meat and that most prized animal flesh – wild game. The table is a tapestry of antipasti: the freshest seafood salad, fished from the Tyrrhenian Sea this very day; *baccalà*, rehydrated and cooked on the grill; and vegetables old and new – preserved peppers and aubergines, new-season artichokes prepared two different ways, celery fritters fried simply in olive oil. It takes an hour to exhaust our taste for these appetizers, and there are four or more courses still to come.

The pasta is thick ribbons of egg-rich *pappardelle* slicked with a *ragù* combining wild boar and wild hare, meats held in reserve for *feste* such as this. We nod our pleasure to Erminia, the guest who made the pasta, and to her husband, who brought the game home to her kitchen.

In the hearth, charcoal smoulders its orange breath onto a grill pan of lamb; the meat spits a response laced with rosemary, garlic and white wine. We eat it hot off the fire, smoky and sweet, like the red wine Adalgesia's husband, Elio, grew on the pergola just metres across the farmyard.

Now it's time for the *lenticchie con cotechino*, the mustiness of the lentils cut by the sweet softness of the pork.

Then a pause before the fruit course of mandarins so fresh they might have been hanging in the citrus groves of nearby Fondi just hours ago.

We're fast approaching the moment for which we are here. So the *prosecco* is popped, froth fills the glasses and we count down the seconds . . . *tre*, *due*, *uno* . . . and *auguri*, best wishes, for the new year.

It arrives with the moonless dark. And I am driving upwards, upwards through the night. Familiar bends on a once-strange road. Into the sleeping village I discovered by chance, and which I now call home.

On the valley-view piazza remain a handful of souls; 'Pina and Attilio serve *prosecco* and panettone at the Moonlight Café. Best wishes and kisses, and now everyone is heading home.

But I linger a while, at the edge of the piazza, where the mountain drops sharp to the valley floor. As I've done so many times, on spring mornings and summer evenings, or whipped by the wind on autumn days. Here I've studied apricot suns setting over purple mountains until the stars pushed through the darkling sky; gazed at moons like lanterns lifted into the night by a hand we cannot see.

But in this first hour of the new year, there's only tumbling darkness studded with occasional house lights – touchstones to guide a traveller's way.

I think of other New Years I have known. Celebrations amid the hustle of big cities and the dazzle of festive lights; midnight moments when I could divine nothing of what the coming year would bring, or the rhythms that would dictate my life. Because in the city, the rhythms are hard to hear.

But here there is a different sense, one of certainty. Because the pattern of the year to come is already known. It's set by the seasons and the sun and the phases of the moon. By the farming calendar and the festivals of the Church. These form the irresistible rhythm to which life is lived. Woven in between will be melodies yet unknown – new lives and joy; death and pain. And the understanding that each has its place, that everything will pass, that the heartbeat of Nature will again make itself felt – uncontrollable and reliable, both at once.

These are the truths that have lived for centuries here, but that can go unheard amid the urban buzz. They are the certainties that give farmers the faith to sow their fields, because they believe the harvest will come; that lead them to stockpile Nature's gifts, because they know lean days must be expected too; that inspire them to give thanks for the food on the table, and to celebrate at the festivals that punctuate the year.

Ogni cosa ha il suo momento. Everything has its moment. Be that person or beast or plant. Acceptance of this wisdom is easy in Campodimele, where Nature sings. And where for many, that moment is longer than for most.

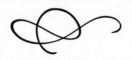

Sedano fritto – Celery fritters

100g (3½oz) '00' Doppio Zero flour or plain white flour
200ml (7fl oz) light beer
One fresh organic egg, beaten
Three or four splashes of extra-virgin olive oil
Fine sea salt
Two large handfuls of celery leaves, roughly chopped, and two
  sticks of celery, cut into 6cm (3in) batons and squashed, to
  break their fibrous spines

Mix the flour and beer in a bowl then beat in the egg, a splash of olive oil and a few pinches of salt.

Add the celery leaves and batons, and coat them well in the batter.

Heat two or three splashes of olive oil in the pan then fry the celery batons for a couple of minutes on each side, until they are swollen and golden.

Next drop spoonfuls of the celery-leaf fritters into the pan, flatten and fry for a minute or two on each side, until golden and cooked through. Serve the fritters hot or at room temperature.

Makes around ten batons.

Cavolfiore alla parmigiana –
Cauliflower fried in Parmesan

Small cauliflower, cut into florets
Three fresh organic eggs
200g (7oz) Parmigiano-Reggiano or Pecorino Romano,
*   finely grated*
Handful of fresh flat-leaf parsley, finely chopped
Fine sea salt
100g (3½oz) '00' Doppio Zero flour or plain white
*   flour*
Seven or eight splashes of extra-virgin olive oil

Bring a large pan of well-salted water to the boil. Add the cauliflower florets to the pan, and let them simmer for around four minutes – or for six minutes if you prefer your cauliflower without bite.

In a large bowl, beat the eggs and mix in the grated cheese, the parsley and a scant pinch of salt.

When the cauliflower is parboiled, drain it into a colander and allow it to steam for a few minutes.

Place the flour in a bowl and lightly dust each of the cauliflower florets with the flour.

Now add the cauliflower to the egg, cheese and parsley mixture, and gently mix with your hands, to ensure all the cauliflower is well coated in the mixture.

Heat three or four splashes of oil in a broad-based frying pan, lower the heat, and add half the cauliflower florets. Fry them gently for four or five minutes, turning constantly, until they are golden all over.

Remove the cauliflower fritters and leave them to cool on a plate lined with kitchen paper, to soak up excess oil.

Clean the frying pan to get rid of any bits of burnt cheese then heat the remainder of the olive oil and fry the rest of the cauliflower in the same way.

Serve the fritters warm, or at room temperature.

Makes around twenty pieces.

Lenticchie con cotechino – Lentils with pig's-snout sausage

The Castelluccio lentils from Lombardy are arguably the best in Italy and they are now widely available outside the country. Fresh *cotechino* sausage can be more difficult to come by, but many precooked and packaged brands are exported, and are often stocked in good Italian delis.

600g (1lb 5oz) cotechino
300g (11oz) green lentils
Three splashes of extra-virgin olive oil
One large golden onion, very finely chopped
One stick of celery, very finely chopped
Two large cloves of garlic, finely chopped (optional)
Handful of fresh flat-leaf parsley, very finely chopped
100g (3½oz) pancetta, finely chopped
Large glass of dry white wine
500ml (1 pint) fresh chicken stock (optional)
Fine sea salt

If using fresh *cotechino*, pierce it all over with a sharp knife then wrap tightly in aluminium foil.

Fill a large, deep pan with just enough water to cover the *cotechino*, bring to the boil then lower the heat and set it to simmer for around two hours. Once it is thoroughly cooked, set aside to rest for ten minutes before unwrapping.

If using precooked *cotechino*, cook according to the instructions on the packaging.

About an hour before your *cotechino* is fully cooked, start preparing the lentils.

Rinse the lentils in cold water, picking out any bits of grit, and leave to drain in a colander.

Heat three splashes of olive oil in a large, deep frying pan then add the onion and celery, and fry gently for around ten minutes, ensuring the onions do not brown.

Add the garlic and parsley, and fry for just a minute.

Next, add the pancetta, and fry for a further minute, stirring frequently.

Now add the lentils and gently mix so they are thoroughly combined with the vegetables. Heat gently for a minute or so, stirring to ensure the lentils do not stick to the bottom of the pan.

Now add the wine, stir well, and raise the heat until the wine bubbles. Continue cooking until the wine is reduced by about half.

If using fresh chicken stock, add enough to the pan to cover the lentils by just 1 cm (½in) – if not using stock, add water in the same way. Return to the boil then lower the heat, cover, and allow the lentils to simmer.

The lentils will absorb the cooking liquid quickly, so check them every ten minutes or so and add more stock or water as required, ensuring that they remain covered at all times. Stir frequently.

Simmer for about forty minutes to an hour, until the lentils are al dente. Then add three or four good pinches of sea salt to taste, and stir well.

Now unwrap the cooked and rested *cotechino* and cut into slices. Create a bed of lentils on a large, warmed serving platter, arrange overlapping slices of the *cotechino* on top, and serve immediately.

Serves six to eight.

Agnello alla cacciatora alla brace –
Lamb with rosemary, garlic and white wine over charcoal

While every region has its own version of the huntsman's pot, in Campodimele '*alla cacciatora*' means meat marinated in rosemary, onion and white wine, and, for those who prefer it, garlic. The style is used for many meats and is possibly my favourite recipe from the village.

1.5kg (3lb 5oz) lamb cutlets, on the bone
One large golden onion, finely sliced
Four cloves of garlic, peeled and squashed by the side of a knife
Two sprigs of fresh rosemary
Large glass of good dry white wine
Extra-virgin olive oil
Fine sea salt

At least twelve hours before you want to eat the lamb, place it in a large bowl with the onion, garlic, rosemary and white wine, and leave to marinate in the fridge, stirring occasionally to ensure the flavours are equally distributed.

The marinated lamb can be cooked *alla brace*, that's to say barbecued, or oven-roasted, if you prefer.

If cooking *alla brace*, set branches to burn around an hour or more ahead of cooking, so they reduce to charcoal.

About forty minutes before you want to eat the cutlets, remove them from the fridge and allow them to return to room temperature.

To cook *alla brace*, remove the meat from the bowl and pat dry with kitchen paper. Brush with a little olive oil, season with a little salt, sandwich into a barbecue grill, and situate beside the charcoal, cooking for around two minutes on each side, depending on the thickness of the lamb.

If you don't have an open wood fire or barbecue, place the lamb in a roasting tin along with the onion, garlic, rosemary and white wine, and cook in an oven preheated to 200°C/400°F/Gas Mark 6 for around thirty minutes, until it is cooked, but still pink inside.

Serves six.

Croccante – Almond crackling

Croccante is sometimes called '*il Torrone dei poveri*' – 'the Torrone of the poor' – Torrone being the nut-rich nougat typical of northern Italy, which is eaten throughout the country during the festive period as part of the sweet course of a meal. This 'poor' substitute is delicious and easy to make at home.

250g (9oz) sweet almonds
3 dsstsp cold water
6 dsstsp white caster sugar

Line a shallow baking tray with greaseproof paper.

Lightly smash the almonds by placing them in a poly-thene bag, sealing it and passing a rolling pin over it.

Place the water in a small, deep pan along with the sugar and heat gently without stirring, until the mixture turns into a rich, golden caramel syrup – this mix can burn easily, so be sure to remove it from the heat before it does.

When the syrup is ready and off the heat, tip in the smashed almonds, stir well then quickly tip the mixture into the shallow baking tray. Spread it in a thin layer and allow it to cool.

Once cooled, the *croccante* should form a stiff sheet, punctuated by the nuts. Cover with another sheet of grease-proof paper and crack into small, bite-size pieces by pressing the blunt end of a rolling pin onto the *croccante*. Store in an airtight container.

Makes about 400g crackling.

The Italian Table – Glossary

'*Sappiamo vivere*', say the Italians – 'we know how to live'. And an integral part of knowing how to live well is knowing how to eat well. Nowhere is that more evident than in Campodimele, where the food is grown, harvested, prepared, eaten and conserved with appreciation and reverence.

Like many Italians, the people of Campodimele tend to eat their main meal of the day at lunchtime, in the form of a leisurely two-hour sitting at the table. This highly civilized tradition persists in the modern age thanks to the fact that schools and many state sector offices end their day between 1.00 p.m. and 2.00 p.m., and many shops – even in central Rome – shut their doors after midday, reopening at around 4.00 p.m.

Traditionally, this workaday lunch has taken the form of a carbohydrate-rich *primo*, which translates as 'first', of pasta, risotto or gnocchi, often dressed in a simple vegetable sauce. This is followed by the *secondo*, which translates as 'second', featuring the protein-rich dish of beans or pulses in the *cucina povera* of the past, or meat or fish in these easier times. The *secondo* is accompanied by the *contorno*, the side dish of vegetables. There follows the *insalata*, a salad often comprising simple green leaves and dressed with olive oil and vinegar, designed to cleanse the palate ahead of the *formaggio*, the cheese which might be nibbled by those with appetite to spare. After that comes the *frutta*, fruit, which is usually fresh from the orchard and seasonal.

This traditional pattern of *primo*, *secondo* with *contorno*, *insalata*, *formaggio*, *frutta* would be preceded at a more celebratory lunch by *antipasti* – which translates as 'before the pasta', and refers to the variety of appetizers such as olives, *salumi*, and out-of-season savoury preserves eaten ahead of the *primo*. This more lavish meal would often feature a *dolce*, or sweet, after the fruit course, perhaps accompanied by a glass of *prosecco*, the Italian sparkling wine.

Drinks are also a key feature of Italian meals – even an everyday lunch might well be preceded by an *aperitivo*, an aperitif at the local bar. Red or white wine and water accompany the meal – and almost all Italians round off lunch with *un bel caffè* – a good coffee.

This pattern of eating at a single sitting may seem unusual to start with – but if you are able to eat like this, do, and you will discover how naturally the meal flows, how civilized lunch becomes, why the Italians can rightly say, '*Sappiamo vivere!*'

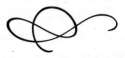

a chi piace – as you like it or, more literally, 'to whom it pleases'.

agrodolce – bitter-sweet, the taste contrast in foods like *amarena* jam, which is a melding of bitter *amarena* cherries and sugar.

al dente – literally translates as 'to the tooth' – pasta should be cooked only to the point where there remains a little bite.

al fresco – in the open air – the beautiful summers of Campodimele make eating outdoors a pleasure.

alimentari – small grocery shop which stocks staple dry goods along-side a fresh deli counter selling an often impressive range of cooked meats and *salumi*, cheeses, marinated olives, grilled vegetables, fresh buffalo mozzarella and a range of breads. Usually independently owned, these stores can still be found on every street corner of Italian towns and live or die according to the quality of their stock, which is therefore often astonishingly good.

alla brace – cooked over charcoal which is created from branches burned down in the open hearth of the kitchen, similar to a barbecue technique.

alla griglia – cooked over an open flame, barbecued.

all' occhio – by eye. This phrase is often an Italian cook's response to the question of how much of a particular ingredient should be included in a recipe, and reflects the idea that the experienced eye can guess accurately.

amarene – small, bitter cherries popular for deliciously tart jam.

antipasti – literally 'before the pasta', a selection of savoury appetizers enjoyed ahead of the pasta at celebratory or special meals.

aroma di limone – extract of lemon oil. Widely available in Italian shops in small glass phials, this can be used in place of lemon zest to add a citrus flavour to cakes and desserts.

artigianale – artisanal – used to describe food products created using traditional methods.

asparago selvatico – wild asparagus.

baccalà – air-dried cod preserved in salt, which is bathed in several changes of water for at least twenty-four hours to rehydrate and desalinate it prior to cooking.

bagnomaria – Italian for the French term *bain-marie*, also known as a double boiler.

besciamella – Italian for the French term *sauce béchamel* – a white sauce of flour, butter and milk, sometimes used in lasagne.

bietola – Swiss chard leafy greens.

biologico – organic. This is a term I have never heard a Campomelano person use, because *biologico* methods of production are the age-old norm in the village.

borgo – the medieval heart of centuries-old Italian villages and small towns – *borgo* generally describes the area which lies within the settlement's defensive walls.

bottiglia – literally translated as 'the bottle', *la bottiglia* is shorthand for the glass bottles full of tomato sauce conserved at home during the tomato glut at the end of every summer.

broccoletti – *rapini* or *cime di rapa* – a leafy edible green widely cultivated in southern Italy, with spiky green leaves and small florets which have a mild almond taste.

brodo – broth, in particular broth or stock created by boiling a chicken with herbs and vegetables. Pasta can be cooked in *brodo* instead of boiling water, to create a tasty *primo*.

bruschetta – slices of toasted bread, usually dressed with olive oil and topped with a variety of toppings including tomato and basil, or just a sprinkling of oregano.

caccialepre – a green salad leaf which grows wild on the mountain-sides surrounding Campodimele, its name translates as something along the lines of 'chase the hare'.

cannella – cinnamon.

cantina – cellar or wine cellar. In Italy the *cantina* is usually a cool, dark place, where conserved foods are stored in order to last the whole year through. Conserving gluts of fresh produce and storing it in the *cantina*, so that it can be eaten throughout the year to come, is pivotal to Campodimele's culinary culture. *Cantina* is also the word used for shops in Italy which sell wine straight from the wine vat to consumers – these are usually an excellent source of good wines at incredibly low prices.

cappuccio – this means 'hood', and is also a name given to a round-bodied, soft-leaved lettuce.

capra – goat.

caprettone – Campomelano dialect for 'young goat'.

carciofi, *carciofini* – globe artichokes and baby globe artichokes.

carne – red meat such as beef and veal.

carne dei poveri – literally 'the meat of the poor', this is the phrase used for beans and pulses which traditionally provided protein in the diet of the poor farming classes who could not afford meat.

casereccio – home-made.

cavolo nero – literally 'black cabbage' – large, dark-leafed cabbages.

centro storico – historic centre. In Campodimele this is the area within the village's defensive walls, which dates from medieval times.

cestini – little cheese moulds, used to form fresh cheese and ricotta.

ciammotte – Campodimele dialect for 'wild snails'.

cibo genuino – 'genuine food'. This simple translation belies the all-encompassing food philosophy behind these words. *Cibo genuino* is food which is grown with respect for the environment, the produce itself and the person who will consume it. It implies an absence of chemicals and industrial processes.

cicerchia – the small pulse particular to Campodimele, once the mainstay of its *cucina povera* and today the focus of an annual street *sagra* in August.

cicoria – 'chicory greens' are a leafy green vegetable with a slightly bitter tang. Not to be confused with chicory – the word used in the UK for Belgian endive.

cime di rapa – see *broccoletti*.

colomba pasquale – the Easter dove, signifying the Holy Spirit in Christian symbology. In culinary terms the *colomba pasquale* is a rich sponge cake, originating from Milan and shaped like a dove, which today is eaten throughout Italy at Easter.

condimenti – condiments. In Campodimele condiments include olive oil, which is used as a dressing as well as a cooking medium, and salt and crushed dried red chilli pepper.

contadino – a person who works the land to grow food for their own consumption. *Contadino* is often translated into English as 'peasant farmer' but the English phrase evokes nothing of the dignity and satisfaction of the *contadino* life. *Fare il contadino* might mean that you earn your living and all you eat from the land, or that you work a vegetable patch outside your home to grow some of your food.

contorno – side dish. The *contorno* is the vegetable accompaniment to the *secondo* course of the meal.

coralli – the word used in Campodimele and the surrounding towns to describe helda beans – stringless green beans that are broad, flat and long in shape.

cotto – cooked – in particular something which has been oven-baked such as *prosciutto cotto*, roast ham.

crispino – a green salad leaf which grows wild on the mountainsides surrounding Campodimele.

crostata – pastry-based tart, usually denoting a jam tart.

crudo – raw or uncooked.

cucina – kitchen. *Cucina* is the word used both for the room in the house where the cooking is done, and to describe the food culture of a particular area – much as the French use the word *cuisine*.

cucina abitabile – translates as 'habitable kitchen'. Still the most desirable room in any Italian home, the *cucina abitabile* denotes a kitchen where the inhabitants can cook, eat around a large dining table and live out the rest of the evening, often with the help of an open fire and the family TV.

cucina povera – literally 'poor kitchen', the phrase used when talking about the traditional cooking of the peasant farming classes during the lean years of the past. This was a culinary culture rich in fruit, vegetables, carbohydrates and beans and pulses, but low in meat and other animal produce.

culo del pane – a polite translation of this would be 'the bottom of the bread' – the curved crusty end of a bread loaf, which might be added stale to soups, toasted to create *bruschetta*, or stuffed with oil-bathed vegetables to create a substantial sandwich.

della zona – literally 'from the zone' – grown locally, as opposed to *casereccio*, which means 'home-grown'.

dolce – dessert or sweet eaten after a meal.

Doppio Zero – literally 'double zero', this is Italy's famous '00' flour – fine-ground white flour sieved not once, but twice by the miller. It creates a strong, smooth dough which is resistant to tearing and so ideal for creating lasagne leaves, though it's also a good all-round baking flour.

fagioli – cannellini beans.

fagiolini – long green beans – called French beans by the British.

fave – broad beans, which are regarded as the first sign of spring in Capodimele and Rome.

festa – party, celebration. *Festa* is the generic word used to signify religious celebrations such as Easter and Christmas as well as birthdays and any other kind of party.

finocchietti – wild fennel seeds.

fiordilatte – cow's milk mozzarella (see *mozzarella fiordilatte*).

formaggi – cheese. As well as describing cheese made from milk solids, this word can be used as a generic term and denotes the cheese course of an Italian meal.

forno a legna – wood-fired oven.

frantoi – olive mills, where olives are crushed to produce olive oil.

frutta verdura – this translates literally as 'fruit vegetables' and is the name given to shops or market stalls which specialize in fresh fruit and vegetables.

fuoco – literally meaning 'fire', this term is also used to describe the gas flame of domestic cooking appliances.

galline – hens. In Campodimele *le galline* is local shorthand for the road which runs along the eastern flank of the village where the hen houses are situated. The term is also a time of day – '*dopo le galline*' or 'after the hens' being used to indicate the hour just after the hens are put to bed – any time from 4.00 p.m. to 6.00 p.m., depending on the time of year and natural daylight.

insalata – salad – used to describe all kinds of composed salads, but in particular the mix of green leaves eaten raw after the *secondo*, or main course of an Italian meal, to refresh the palate. *Insalata* is also the generic word for lettuce.

in umido – stewed, cooked over heat in liquid, usually with a pan which has a lid on.

iper-mediterraneo – hyper-Mediterranean – a term used to describe the Campomelano diet, which is an extreme example of the traditional Mediterranean diet.

laine – the traditional pasta ribbons of Campodimele, made from just flour and water – as opposed to *pasta all'uovo*, which is made from flour and eggs, and is richer and traditionally eaten on special occasions.

laine e fagioli – a signature dish of Campodimele, this consists of the flour-and-water pasta ribbons of *laine*, dressed in a sauce of cannellini beans which usually has a tomato base.

legumi – legumes, including beans, peas and lentils and the *cicerchia*, which is particular to Campodimele.

lievito naturale – 'natural leavening' – sourdough leavening which contains only yeasts found in the air and flour – without any brewer's yeast.

livio – a farming tool used to thresh foods which have dried on the plant, such as *cicerchie* or *fagioli*. Made from two branches loosely held together by a flexible leather hinge.

luna calante – waning moon – as opposed to the crescent, or growing moon. According to folklore, *la luna calante* is regarded as the ideal time to sow and reap crops in Campodimele.

magazzino – an outdoor storehouse, more likely to be used for non-food items, as opposed to the *cantina* which is where conserved food, wine and olive oil are usually stored.

maiale – pork, often referring to pork fillet.

maniella – Campomelano dialect for a large, deep wooden tray with a handle at each corner, used in the preparation of large quantities of food, such as mixing the ingredients to make bread dough.

melanzane – aubergines, also known as eggplants. The word *melanzana* is said to derive from the Italian *mela insana*, or 'mad apple', because aubergines were once believed to cause insanity.

mescolata – beautifully onomatopoeic Campomelano word to describe giving a pan full of ingredients a thorough mix with a wooden spoon.

millefoglie – puff-pastry cake or dessert.

minestra – mixed vegetable soup, often including beans in the mix.

mosca dell'olivo – the olive fly, a pest which can ravage olive crops.

mozzarella di bufala – mozzarella cheese made with milk from domesticated water buffalos. This mozzarella is at its best eaten the day it is made and uncooked in salads, such as tomato, mozzarella and basil salad.

mozzarella fiordilatte – mozzarella cheese made from fresh cow's milk. Cow's milk mozzarella is less moist than *mozzarella di bufala* (above) and so is more suitable for cooking, and is often used to top dishes such as lasagne. It is often sold pre-packaged, and will last for several days in the fridge.

mulino per verdure – a hand-operated kitchen device through which *verdure*, vegetables, are passed in order to purée them. Also used to create *passata* – the thick tomato sauce whose name translates literally as 'passed'.

mungitura – the milking of cows or goats or other animals.

odori – the herbs and other foods used to add flavour to a dish. The classic *odori* of the Campodimele *cucina* are very finely chopped celery, parsley and golden onions – or celery, parsley and garlic. Most Campomelano cooks use only onions or garlic in any single dish – few mix both.

orto – domestic vegetable garden or orchard.

pancetta – salt-cured pork from the underbelly of the pig.

pane al forno a legna – bread baked in a wood-fired oven.

panettone – the dome-shaped, rough-textured sponge cake believed to have originated in Lombardy and which has become the traditional Christmas cake throughout Italy.

pappardelle – ribbons of pasta, made from *pasta all'uovo*, fresh egg pasta, and served dressed in a meat sauce.

Parmigiano-Reggiano – world-famous hard cheese made from cow's milk, known as Parmesan in the UK and US. Originating from the north, this cheese is widely available throughout Italy, and grated and scattered on pasta dishes. This is one northern import which has made some inroads in Campodimele, although a hard pecorino, or sheep's cheese made locally, or the more famous *Pecorino Romano*, much of which is made in Sardinia, is often used in its place.

passata – literally 'passed', this refers to tomato sauce which has been passed through a *mulino per verdure*, a hand-operated vegetable mill, to reduce the sauce to a smooth, purée-like consistency and to eliminate skin and seeds.

passeggiata – the *passeggiata* is the evening walk traditionally taken by Italians before and sometimes after dinner – usually down to the piazza to catch up with friends and family.

pasta – literally meaning 'paste' or 'dough', this word is used to describe the full range of culinary doughs, including those for bread and pastry. It is also the generic term for the mix of flour, water and sometimes eggs used to make the range of pastas such as spaghetti and lasagne.

pasta all' uovo – pasta made with eggs and flour as opposed to water and flour. Used to create richer pastas like lasagne leaves and tagliatelle, which are reserved for dishes on celebratory days when it is likely to be dressed with a meat sauce.

Pecorino Romano – hard cheese made from ewe's milk, this is often used as an alternative to *Parmigiano-Reggiano* cheese. Grated and scattered over pasta, a little goes a long way. This cheese is made in a number of areas, including Sardinia and parts of Tuscany.

peperoncino – hot chilli pepper, the staple seasoning in Campodimele.

peperoncino rosso – red hot chilli pepper.

peperoncino rotondo – round-bellied hot chilli pepper.

peperoncino verde – green hot chilli pepper.

pesci azzurri – 'azure fish' – the term Italians use to describe oily fish such as sardines.

petartela – Campomelano dialect for finely ground coriander seeds, used to help flavour and preserve the air-dried, home-made sausage traditionally made from the family pig in Campodimele every January.

piccante – literally 'stinging'. Used to describe spicy food, particularly food laced with red chilli pepper.

pignatta – hand-thrown ceramic jug with two loop-handles. The *pignatta* is particular to the Campodimele area and is commonly used to slow-cook *cicerchie* and beans beside an open fire.

pilosella – a wild green leaf, gathered and eaten in green salads.

pinzimonio – a dish of raw vegetables which are served along with olive oil, salt and pepper seasonings. Dipped in the oil and seasonings, the crudités are popular antipasti.

prezzemolo – parsley.

primo – the first course, which translates literally as 'first'.

prosciutto – air-dried ham, usually served in wafer-thin slices.

prosecco – Italian sparkling wine, generally cheaper but often just as delicious as French sparkling wines.

ragù – meat sauce, traditionally served with pasta.

rapini – see *broccoletti*.

ricotta – soft, white, fresh cheese, which can be made from the milk of goats, sheep, cows or water buffalo – and often in Italy from a combination of these. *Ricotta* translates literally as 'recooked' and is so named because it is made from the solids which rise to the surface when the whey of the milk is heated for a second time – solids from the first heating of the whey being used for the *formaggio*, cheese.

roba nostra – our own things, used to describe home-grown fresh produce.

sagra – a local festival, often held in honour of a particular food, just as the harvest is gathered in.

salsa verde – 'green sauce'. As a rule, *salsa verde* in Italy refers to a green herb sauce made from a combination of parsley, capers, garlic, anchovies, vinegar and olive oil and served as an accompaniment to meat or fish. However the *salsa verde* of Campodimele is a combination of mint and garlic, and is the traditional cooking sauce for the snails served to celebrate the religious *festa* of San Onofrio, one of the patron saints of Campodimele.

salsicce – air-cured sausages, such as those traditionally home-made in Campodimele from the family pig in January.

salsiccia dolce – non-spicy sausage.

salsiccia fresca – fresh sausage, made to be eaten and cooked within a day or so of making.

salsiccia piccante – spicy sausage, usually containing hot chilli pepper and perhaps ground coriander.

salumi – generic term for air-cured and cooked meats.

scalogni – shallots.

scarola – lettuce with spiky leaves which is traditionally added to minestrone mixed vegetable soup in the Campodimele area to add a bitter sweetness to the mix.

secondo – the second course of an everyday meal, featuring the main protein dish such as legumes, meat or fish. This is served after the *primo* of pasta and alongside the *contorno* of vegetables.

setaccio – sieve.

sfoglia – sheet of pastry or pasta which has been rolled out.

sfogliatelle – shell-shaped pastries crafted from a filo-type pastry and filled with ricotta which has been flavoured with candied orange then baked. Said to have been created at the Santa Rosa monastery at Conca dei Marini, on Italy's Amalfi coast, these delicious pastries remain a speciality of Naples and the surrounding area, and are at their most delicious eaten warm from the oven and swigged down with a syrupy espresso.

sott'aceto – literally 'under vinegar', this term refers to foods preserved in vinegar so that they will last all year round – such as peppers.

sott'olio – 'under oil', signifying foods which are preserved in olive oil so that they can be stored and enjoyed later in the year.

sotto peso – translated literally as 'under weight', *sotto peso* is a means of forcing water out of produce before cooking or preserving – for example aubergines, which are around 90 per cent water, are sliced and placed in a bowl under a heavy weight for several hours, to ensure all excess water is eliminated prior to preserving under oil.

sottovuoto – vacuum-packed, a modern but non-chemical way of preserving foods which Campomelani are happy to use.

strisciarelle – strips, used to refer to the pastry strips traditionally laid out in a lattice formation on Campomelano tarts.

strutto – pork lard.

sugetto, *sugo* – literally *sugetto* means 'little sauce', while *sugo* means 'sauce'.

sugo bianco – literally 'white sauce' this refers to sauces which do not contain tomatoes, and which often have a base of olive oil and white wine. In my experience *sugo bianco* is not used to denote white sauces such as béchamel sauce.

sugo rosso – literally 'red sauce', this refers to tomato-based sauces, as opposed to a *sugo bianco* which has no tomatoes (see above).

tagliolini – skinny pasta ribbons. Usually made from *pasta all'uovo*, fresh egg pasta, and often served in a *brodo*, a broth created from chicken stock.

tagne – a signature dish of Campodimele, the *tagne* is an egg-free, pan-fried frittata, made from gathered wild greens – *Clematis vitalba*, known in the UK as 'old man's beard' is the favourite. This plant is toxic to human beings, though a relatively low level of toxin is found in the youngest green shoots gathered to make *tagne*, and this dissipates somewhat under heat. Nevertheless, it is not recommended that this plant be eaten in any great quantity.

terreno – land, referring to the land on which food is farmed.

tortano – the Easter sweet particular to Campodimele shaped like a large doughnut and flavoured with wild fennel seeds.

trebbia – combine harvester. *La trebbia* denotes the machine and the wider concept of the wheat harvest itself.

un'altra cosa – another thing, something else – this phrase often implies the sense of a tastier thing, a better thing.

uva – grape.

uva da tavola – 'table grapes', perfect for eating fresh from the vine.

uva fragola – strawberry grape. The small, ruby-red grape which has the taste and scent of strawberries and is best eaten sun-warmed and fresh from the vine, or mixed with ripe figs to create strawberry grape and fig jam.

uva per vino – grapes for wine-making.

verdure – the generic Italian word for vegetables, *verdure* is most often used in Campodimele to refer to leafy greens which require cooking, such as spinach, chard, cabbage and *cicoria* – chicory greens.

vitello macinato – minced veal, or young beef cattle, used to create a *ragù* for dishes such as lasagne.

zuppa – soup.

zucchina – what the British call a courgette.

List of Recipes

October

November

Acknowledgements

A Year in the Village of Eternity has come to fruition thanks only to the incredible generosity of the people of Campodimele.

The warmth and kindness with which the Campomelani have welcomed me to their village has been truly overwhelming and I will never be able to thank them enough for the friendship and hospitality they have bestowed on me – no matter how long I live!

I would like to thank the people who have led the administration of Campodimele in recent years – Generale Aldo Lisetti, Paolo Zannella and Roberto Zannella, successive mayors of the village and Alessandro Grossi, deputy mayor, who have done so much to help Campodimele flourish as *Il Paese della Longevità*.

But the entire list of individuals to whom I owe thanks is too, too long to feature here – it includes not only the people who feature in this book, but every person who invited me into their *orto*, flung open their larder doors and welcomed me to their table with a hospitality which has been breath-taking – even by Italian standards. And those people who offered a wave or smile or briefly passed the time of day while I sipped an espresso at the piazza's Moonlight Café. And the friends I made in the surrounding towns of Fondi, Lenola, Formia, Sperlonga and Gaeta, with whom I shared such lovely times. Thank you for making me feel so at home in a foreign land.

I know now that my journey to Campodimele started many years before I first set foot in Italy. For this I thank my parents – my mother, Joan, and my late father, George – who opened the world to me through literature and travel, encouraged my love of

languages and allowed my childhood self to believe I wou
write books. Words alone can not thank them for these g.

Thanks also my brother, Michael – and his patience wi
nical support!

Thanks too to my agent, Mark Stanton (Stan) at Jenny Bu
Associates in Edinburgh and to Jenny herself – without their ins
enthusiasm and faith this book might never have been written.

And to everyone at Bloomsbury Publishing – Richard Atkinson,
Natalie Hunt and Xa Shaw Stewart in editorial and Laura Brooke in
publicity. Also Mike Jones, formerly of the editorial department at
Bloomsbury, who championed this book from the very start.
Thanks also to photographer Jason Lowe.

I would also like to say a huge thank you to old friends and
former colleagues who have wished me well in this venture – in
particular Lennox Morrison, Alan Smith and Linda Kennedy, who
assured me this was a book they would love to read, and whose
encouragement sustained me to the very final full stop.